Praise for *The Protector Ethic*

"I knew the book would be good, but the book is actually very good. It breaks new ground, not just for aspiring and practicing martial artists but for anyone who is concerned with—and would like to see a decrease in—human violence. I venture to say there is also much to excite those interested in the intellectual pursuits of philosophy. The book will be helpful for anyone trying to make sense of the natural law in a useful way.

"*The Protector Ethic*, I believe, will ultimately be viewed as one of the most unique and helpful books on martial philosophy ever written. And, as an added benefit, it is a very entertaining read."

—Jack Hoban (from his foreword), president,
Resolution Group International LLC; author,
The Ethical Warrior

"James Morganelli is a gifted and inspirational leader and martial artist who has a strong legacy of service to our country using the ethics of being a protector. This book is an invitation to the simple understanding of the protector mind-set designed for self-improvement as a martial artist and, more importantly, as an ethical protector of self and all others. As you examine this mind-set in relation to yourself and your actions every day, you will become a stronger, more ethical person in everything you do. And as you take this concept on board and change for the better, so shall all those around you."

—Joseph C. Shusko, marine (retired); director,
Marine Corps Martial Arts Program; author, *Tie-Ins for Life*

"A martial artist of both the physical and verbal ilk, James Morganelli has written a complex and yet uplifting book defending what he terms a 'protector ethic'—an ethic that uniquely yokes mental and bodily practice. Choc-a-bloc with compelling personal stories and ethical analysis, Mr. Morganelli's work is a bracing call to duty, the duty never to close the shades when the golem of injustice is working someone over outside our window. It is a heartfelt and well-argued reflection that will appeal to all aspiring Good Samaritans."

—Dr. Gordon Marino, boxing trainer; author,
The Existentialist Survival Guide

"The highest accomplishment in Japanese martial arts is the state transcending all conflict and division called *muteki*, 'no-enemy.' In the *Hagakure*, it is famously said that a warrior must outwardly manifest fearlessness, but inwardly cultivate compassion to the point that one's heart nearly bursts.

"It is in the spirit of these profound principles that James Morganelli Sensei asks a question with which we all must grapple: How, in this world indeed marked by conflict and division, is one to live with integrity, honor, and caretaking for others? Those who take up the study of martial skills, whether as a *way* of personal refinement, a method to preserve life, in the actual profession of arms, or all of these, must consider this with particular care. *The Protector Ethic*, revealing Morganelli Sensei's own deep examination of such questions over many years of training, will surely become a valued resource for those walking a martial path."

—Meido Moore, abbot, Korinji Rinzai Zen Monastery;
sixth dan, aikido; author, *The Rinzai Zen Way*

"In a world overwhelmed with information and conflicting values, James Morganelli's book *The Protector Ethic* dives deep beneath the surface of superficial technique to clarify the essence of true martial arts training and what it means to be a protector. The message James's book presents is essential not only for the martial artist but for *anyone* who has ever been in conflict with another human being."

—Craig Gray, conflict-management consultant;
krav maga and defensive tactics instructor

"Wow, a truly exceptional read. James has a tremendous amount of experience within this field of study, which makes him a great deliverer for his message. The book is factual, funny, and at times extremely inspirational. As a retired detective for the NYPD, I can see how useful the content in this extremely well-written book can be for all law enforcement officers throughout the world."
—Arthur D. Mark, detective (retired), NYPD;
Shihan sixth dan, Okinawan Shorinji Arashiryu

"I feel privileged for this opportunity to support and endorse this valuable work by my friend and colleague, James V. Morganelli. I can attest to his status as a genuine teacher, practitioner, and authentic subject-matter expert on the contents of this remarkable book. He possesses both the creativity and credibility to foster the unique amalgamation of esoteric Eastern martial arts philosophy and complex Western psychological theory. It is clearly and generously presented in a practical fashion and makes for easy assimilation for the novice as well as the established adherent in this field. This book will find a place of honor in my personal library, and I will advocate for its use by my students. In conclusion, I wish the author all the good things a man of his integrity and vitality deserves."
—James T. Shanahan, detective (retired),
NYPD; founder, NYPD Police Academy
and Hostage Negotiation Team; chief instructor,
Keisatsu Dojo, LLC

"With *The Protector Ethic*, Morganelli has given us three books. This is a book for people interested in ethics, who want to know what they can do to make the world a better place—train!
"This is a book for martial artists who want to explore the reason for training and its foundations. Why train? To protect life!

"But most important, this is a book for people who haven't yet realized how these two points—the martial and the moral—are connected, and how important that is."

—Jason G. Cather, PhD; adjunct professor of philosophy, Saint Xavier University; fifth dan, Bujinkan

THE PROTECTOR ETHIC

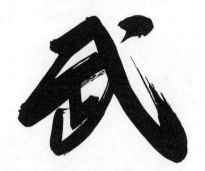

THE
PROTECTOR
ETHIC

Morality, Virtue, and Ethics
in the Martial Way

JAMES V. MORGANELLI

YMAA Publication Center
Wolfeboro, NH USA

YMAA Publication Center, Inc.
PO Box 480
Wolfeboro, New Hampshire, 03894
1-800-669-8892 • info@ymaa.com • www.ymaa.com

ISBN: 9781594395581 (print) • ISBN: 9781594395598 (ebook)

Edited by T. G. LaFredo
Cover design by Axie Breen
This book typeset in 12 pt. Adobe Garamond.
Typesetting by Westchester Publishing Services
10 9 8 7 6 5 4 3 2 1

Publisher's Cataloging in Publication

Names: Morganelli, James V., author.
Title: The protector ethic : morality, virtue, and ethics in the martial way / James V. Morganelli.
Description: Wolfeboro, NH USA : YMAA Publication Center, Inc., [2018] | Includes bibliographical references.
Identifiers: ISBN: 9781594395581 (print) | 9781594395598 (ebook) | LCCN: 2017963167
Subjects: LCSH: Martial artists—Conduct of life. | Martial arts—Moral and ethical aspects. | Martial arts—Psychological aspects. | Hand-to-hand fighting, Oriental—Philosophy. | Violence—Moral and ethical aspects. | Violence—Psychological aspects. | Self-defense—Moral and ethical aspects. | Discipline—Moral and ethical aspects. | Justice—Moral and ethical aspects. | Vigilance (Psychology) | Courage—Moral and ethical aspects. | BISAC: SPORTS & RECREATION / Martial Arts & Self-Defense. | PHILOSOPHY / Ethics & Moral Philosophy. | PHILOSOPHY / Good & Evil.
Classification: LCC: GV1102.7.P75 M674 2018 | DDC: 796.815—dc23

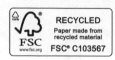

To my wife,
who is my protector

The nation that will insist on drawing a broad line of demarcation between the fighting man and the thinking man is liable to find its fighting done by fools and its thinking done by cowards.

—Sir William Francis Butler, *Charles George Gordon* (1889)

Contents

Foreword

WHEN JAMES TOLD ME he was writing *The Protector Ethic: Morality, Virtue, and Ethics in the Martial Way*, I was very happy. Partially, this was because he is a good writer and he should write. But most importantly, he is an expert on the subject matter—the ethics of the protector. This expertise comes from years of hard work and sacrifice in the physical disciplines of the martial arts, as well as in the intellectual rigors of formal ethics training and study.

I knew the book would be good, but the book is actually very good. It breaks new ground, not just for aspiring and practicing martial artists but for anyone who is concerned with—and would like to see a decrease in—human violence. I venture to say there is also much to excite those interested in the intellectual pursuits of philosophy. The book will be helpful for anyone trying to make sense of the natural law in a useful way.

The other value of this book is that it represents a fresh bridge between Eastern and Western philosophical thought. Particularly in America, we consider our martial prowess to be a hallmark. It is not. Our prowess is technology and resources, mixed with a little stubbornness and topped off with an organic moral sense inherited from our founders. Our martial philosophy is deeply flawed, as can be seen in the frightening numbers of American warriors who come back from their combat-related experiences with psychological and moral injuries.

The shortcomings of Eastern politics are self-evident, but the philosophical strengths of Asian martial thought are a treasure still to be mined. James does the mining in the context of Robert L. Humphrey's astoundingly satisfying Dual-Life Value theory of human nature. James makes sense of the often less-than-literal nature of Eastern thought in a way that the reader will find new and worthwhile. When East meets West in this book, the reader sees that life is the superseding, absolute value that all humans share, regardless of culture or ethnicity, and that our ethical imperative is to protect life. Whose life? Self and others. Which others? All others.

And that is what the martial arts represent—a skill set to bring into action our intrinsic moral inclinations to protect and respect life. If the philosophy of the West can articulate why life is an absolute value, the martial philosophies of the East can teach us how to practice that value as an ethic.

I really believe that the world needs a refresher and clarification on the subject of values, morals, and ethics. And that is why this book is important *now*. And not only for martial artists. It is heartbreaking to see men and women who are supposed to be our leaders and role models in business, government, the military, law enforcement, entertainment, sports, and even religion failing to act morally. This holds dire consequences for the rest of us, not just directly, although we are often physical, political, or economic victims of their lack of ethics. But we are *philosophical* victims as well.

When we see our role models and leaders acting immorally (and succeeding!), we ask ourselves if we might be the patsies. If we may be wrong. We wonder if we should be doing what they are doing. It seems to be the road to success in the world—this world, anyway. They are doing it, so why not us? If we don't do it, someone else will, right? After all, who is to say what's truly right or wrong?

And there you have it: the disease of moral relativism. Modeled by our leaders with a chilling trickle-down effect on us all.

James proposes that we have become a nation (world?) dominated by moral and cultural relativism. *Moral relativism* means that if an attitude or action doesn't directly injure or disrespect "my tribe" (country, race, color, ethnic group, religion, company, team, and so on), then it is OK. Anybody outside our "in-group" is fair game. *Cultural relativism* means that all cultures are equal, just different, and you have to respect all of them. These mutually exclusive concepts, often somehow lumped together, are both dead wrong.

You've heard the phrase "Everything's relative"? Not quite. Almost all values are relative—different for me from how they are for you. But the value of life is not relative; we all share it—those in our tribe and those outside our tribe. Equally. Tribal values are relative; the life value is not.

Don't overthink this—we all have it, or we wouldn't be alive. And if we were not alive, we would have no need for our other values. Some of which involve respecting the life of self and others. Some of which do not. Life, therefore, is not only the absolute value; it is the *superseding* value by which all other, relative, values must be qualified.

James argues that we need not like or respect the relative or cultural values of others, especially those values that are dangerous to those outside our in-groups. But we must value and respect the *life value* of self and others—all others. When we demonize, or dehumanize, those outside our in-group—that is, those who do not share our relative values—we violate the sacred life value. And the conflict, and perhaps violence, and perhaps killing, starts. Guaranteed.

And from this arises James's perception of a warrior. A protector of life. Whose life? Self and others. Which others? All others. Can we separate the relative values of others' beliefs and actions, some of which may be moral, neutral, or immoral, from the absolute value of life and our respect for it? That's the discipline of the warrior. And James clarifies the philosophical basis for this transcending imperative.

James's book, I believe, will ultimately be viewed as one of the most unique and helpful books on martial philosophy ever written. And, as an added benefit, it is a very entertaining read.

Enjoy it, think about what he says, and share the insights with your family and friends.

Jack Hoban, president, Resolution Group International LLC, author of *The Ethical Warrior*

"I'M AT LAUGHING MAN TAVERN in Washington, DC." This is the last tweet of Kevin Joseph Sutherland. It's dated July 3, 2015.

In the early afternoon of July Fourth, Sutherland boards the Metro Red Line to meet friends downtown to watch fireworks. He is twenty-four, has recently graduated from American University, and has been hired as a digital strategist for a DC firm.

Just before 1 p.m. another passenger, eighteen-year-old Jasper Spires, tries to take Sutherland's cell phone. He resists. They tussle. And now it's a beating. Ten other passengers watch.

Spires pulls a pocketknife and stabs Sutherland more than forty times. He stomps him and kicks him. He dropkicks his head and even destroys the phone he originally tried to steal, smashing it against Kevin's face.

Spires then turns on the others and demands their money. One gives him $65, another $160. He gets off at the next stop. He throws away bloody clothing, the knife, and a book bag containing his ID, and skips past police, who are looking for him.

Sutherland dies on the floor of car 3045. It's the first homicide in the transit system's four decades of existence.

Two days later Spires is arrested and charged with first-degree murder. A crucial piece of evidence: CCTV footage of Sutherland and Spires boarding at Rhode Island Avenue, where the train leaves at 12:46 p.m. It arrives at NoMa–Gallaudet, the very next stop, at 12:49. The attack, murder, and robberies took all of three minutes.

Prologue

When I was nine, Mom enrolled me in karate class. Growing up, I was a small kid and got smacked around some, especially at that age when even nice kids bully just to try it out. I remember my instructor wore a black uniform, so it was probably kempo I was learning, but when I was nine, "karate" was what I called all that stuff.

Twice a week during that summer, we gathered at the rec center in Riverside, Illinois, a quiet hamlet with twisty streets just southwest of Chicago. I don't remember my instructor's name. I do remember he was young and rocked a stache, just like my favorite TV private eye, Thomas Magnum, so I just assumed he had a closet full of Hawaiian shirts and drove a Ferrari.

Those classes stopped once the school year began. As of this writing, I will soon see four decades in martial arts. That may seem like a long time. It's not.

By twenty-one I was prone to extremes. At five eight and a lean 150, I could dive roll over the roof of a hatchback—yes, the roof—break bricks with my hands and feet, and max a bench press of 320 pounds, more than twice my body weight. I was a teetotaler but smoked cigars like somebody bet I wouldn't. And I mouthed off. A lot.

I liked brutal sparring and ultraviolent techniques. The Ultimate Fighting Championship (UFC) was just airing, and was my new favorite thing because it seemed to mash up cartoons and kung fu movies— two of my other favorite things. So when a Russian gongfu expert challenged me to a "match," I knew it was just code for "fight," and I put him down. And a few others along the way. Usually, I was charming enough to get away with poor decisions. But not always, like the night a noise complaint landed me at the business end of Sheriffs' pistols.

I read a lot. Still do. I picked up books like this one, looking for insight. When I graduated from college, I moved to Japan to train and study. When I returned years later, I founded a school to keep training and studying. I earned a master's degree in philosophy. I was still searching. Still am.

Are you seeking ancient martial secrets? Here's one: you already know how to defend yourself. A qualified instructor can run you through the basics, but that can take all of ten minutes. After that the serious work begins to reactivate and refine the instincts we take for granted.

People come to the martial way for all kinds of reasons, some of them good, most of them not good enough. Others have watched too many action movies. A select few seek the supernatural, working hard to sound just like the gongfu master's master whenever they open their mouths, which is often, far too often. Deceit is at its worst when we believe our own lies, so avoid those who talk like Yoda and move like Jabba.

It took years for my own temperament to change, but that's not just my story; it's the life cycle of any serious martial artist. To break the mold of the form and enter the fray of the formless, where the real training takes place, you have to give up looking for answers. Only then can you do what must be done: ask better questions. You have to. Skills like exceptional punching and kicking only improves further once you understand and articulate an ethos for it. So you start with the question most avoid asking because they have a less-than-inspiring answer or, worse, none at all: Why?

Why am I doing this?

Why should I learn any of this stuff?

Why train?

Logic and reasoning can lead that inquiry. Other times a simple story convinces in a way argument cannot. Isn't clarity the point? In fact, clear thinking on big questions begets bigger ones, like resolving right from wrong, deciding action from obligation, and facing up to the musts, oughts, and shoulds. If we're going to use our bodies as weapons, and weapons as weapons, we'd better train our minds to discern wisdom from knowledge so we can act in the right way at the right time. Do this and avoid the worst possible fate, the one where we're too late to make any difference.

Do you agree with the following statement?

I cannot intervene to stop an attack on another person because I am not physically capable.

It's nonsense—claptrap, pretention to illicit approval, a ploy to con our higher sensibilities.

To even think about responding to the terror that struck Kevin Sutherland on the DC Metro line that sunny July day can leave decent folks inert—an utterly normal response, by the way. But dread is hardly an excuse for inaction, since its answer is so predictable—it always favors inertness.

"Agitation and anxiety caused by the presence or imminence of danger"—this is the dictionary definition of fear. But why should danger cause us fear when we do dangerous stuff every day? We slam into each other in hard-charging sports, snapping bones and joints; we enjoy diets full of junk that satisfy but poison us; and, like Pollyanna, we naively turn the privacy of our lives over to the titans of the virtual— and any criminals paying attention—just to buck our anonymity with a megapixel shot of a sushi platter. Driving a car is by far one of the most dangerous things anyone can possibly do. Over a five-year period, more than 25 percent of drivers will be involved in an accident—that's one out of four! If I had a one-out-of-four chance of being eaten by a shark, I wouldn't swim in a backyard pool. So, if danger doesn't scare us, what gives?

People fear death. People fear pain. But nothing causes fear like having to deal with conflict. Human conflict is by far the number one phobia of our species, and most folks will do just about anything to avoid it, including ignoring suffering, cries for mercy, even our own conscience pleading to lend aid. Why do you think there is such a divide in how we view, debate, and carry out our social contracts, cultural beliefs, and politics? It's because ambivalence toward traditional and time-honored mores is pandemic in this twenty-first century and the reason why is simple: most folks are terrified.

To save us, *skepticism*—the doubt that assails the search for truth—cozies up with soft words and bears gifts to transform our fear of conflict into a superficial strength. Some see this as compassionate tolerance and others a kind of civility—a way toward greater equality through the mantra "Different strokes for different folks" or "Live and let live." But it is hardly that. Its true self is masked, and underneath is one of man's oldest foes that holds contempt for the good, cynicism toward the joy of wonder, and a thick suspicion and distrust for truth itself. Its name is *nihilism*.

If nihilism were a person, he would be a supervillain living in a hollowed-out volcano with an army of ninjas waiting to die in his name. Nihilism may seem foreign, but it's quite domestic—all spoiled children, whether children or adults, are nihilists at some point, for it's the malady symptomatic of selfishness and its dearth of gratitude. The nihilistic ideal does not just lead to ethical befuddlement; it leads to moral confusion because it advocates for willful ignorance in the prioritization of values, the principles or standards of our behavior. Not only do we not know what to do ethically, but we don't know why we do not know.

Some values are more important than other values. When we deny that, we're not on top of Mount Righteous waving the banner of tolerance; we're hunting down and culling truth with torches and pitchforks.

Nihilism makes us bystanders, ones who willingly sacrifice the sacred to the senseless and art to the artificial. Choosing to stand for nothing allows the promotion of anything. In fact, when the zeitgeist equates all values, it provides the perfect cover to join in because, hell, everybody's doing it. But this groupthink bears an unintended consequence: it normalizes the sick and twisted. Faced with a zombie apocalypse, rather than fight, we stand shoulder to shoulder with the risen dead as zombie activists, waving signs and yelling, "Zombie rights now!"—just before we're surrounded and devoured.

From behind this veil of equivocation, folks can aspire to a world in which no value is greater because all of them are lesser. Conflict can then only occur when we choose to take a stand. But choose to stand for nothing and you protect you and yours. There are plenty who believe this to be a good, righteous, enlightened view of the world.

They're wrong. It's a joke—a sick and killing one.

The aim of morals, ethics, and especially virtue—the pinnacle of our moral and ethical endeavors—is not to avoid the fight but ensure that it's worth fighting. Denying the causes of conflict does not alleviate but stoke, especially when faced with intolerable values like those that threaten, harm, torture, and murder innocents in the name of culture or creed. Distorting reality through groupthink and manipulating language and popular culture to claim the mantle of the right and the good is to deceive fundamentally on the matter of rightness and goodness. Consensus is never a worthwhile end if it means consensual suicide. Only the ignorant and dishonest are assured there is nothing worth risking themselves for. But this reasoning is as twisty as a Gordian knot. Fidelity to truth is not about unraveling these knots but, like Alexander, cutting them.

Intervention is often underrated in the aftermath of horror, usually by the bystanders who did nothing. It is hard to imagine, however, that these same folks would have discouraged passengers from coming to their own loved one's aid. Would they have asked them politely to stop? Encouraged them to look out for themselves? Do you think Kevin Sutherland appreciated in those last moments the fact that no one dared intercede? After all, these folks only did what normal people think they should normally do: stay out of it.

Hardly.

Our absolute needs become our fiercest desires when we find them in short supply. Just ask anyone saved from drowning. No one is more grateful for a life saved than the saved life.

But try telling that to those who are convinced there is no magnetic north on the moral compass, like the writer at the *Washington Post* who softened the blow of her own nihilism with cooing solidarity: "It makes a lot of us uncomfortable to think we would have cowered instead of confronting Sutherland's killer."[1] Of course it's uncomfortable. It should be. We are all perfectly capable of intervening. *We make a conscious choice not to.*

Everyone has the mental, spiritual, and physical fortitude to intervene on behalf of another who needs protection. Who would be unwilling to shield their child, sibling, or spouse under brutal attack? Those who love them can throw themselves on their bodies to shield them from violence. Anyone mobile is capable of doing this, from Grandma to Junior, and people of all kinds have. No one has to be made of steel to intervene, because doing violence to the aggressor is not the point. Protecting the victim is.

If we do not acknowledge this difference, then we stand to applaud the claptrap and confide in the con that says we are powerless. This is irrational fear, the worst kind, and it seduces into that cult of victimhood—a cult of death—where we expect to be a victim at some point, and our only defense is the condemning hope that sheer numbers safeguard us from being next.

If you're unwilling to risk your life to protect a complete stranger, congratulations, you're a member of the club called *human*. There are plenty of folks—good folks, mind you—who will never bring themselves to intervene. But do not confuse that raw fact of our humanity with the moral, ethical, or virtuous, should, ought, and must.

However, if you are willing to risk yourself to protect others, that makes you above and beyond—superhuman, in fact—and we have a name for those people: heroes. And just so we're clear, those willing to risk their lives to protect the lives of others, *and physically engage attackers to rout them, kill them, or subdue them*, well, we call those rare folks by another name: warriors.

The best that martial training can do is not simply provide the necessary mental and physical skills to respond to conflict, but calibrate ourselves *justly* to know we ought to respond. That's another of those ancient martial secrets. In fact, you will find these secrets have one thing in common: they all concern, touch, and overlap the realm of ethics.

Placing ethics first, ahead of physical, tactical concerns, isn't simply more *difficult* because it requires more training, more study, and skill. It's more *life threatening* because it forces us to risk our lives for ourselves and others and thereby requires greater fortitude of will for the courage to act. Any book can splash photos of techniques across its pages. I admit, this book aspires to something more: to articulate why it is harder, tougher, requires more competence, more strength of character, and more faith in oneself, to be ethical before we are tactical.

The best definition of ethics I ever heard did not come from some inscrutable ancient philosopher or religious exponent or secular concern, although each of these has contributed in some capacity to its historical meaning. It actually came from a US Marine Corps captain, a mentor of mine, who stated that ethics is nothing more than our "moral values in action."

Damn.

The simple and sublime from someone trained to shoot and blow things up. From a man trained to fight.

We ought to protect others. We ought to shield them and defend them if we must, so as to escape threats and violence. And we ought to want to.

Soldiers and police officers are protectors by duty. But so are moms and dads and schoolteachers. So is the pizza guy, the investment banker, and old lady Smith down the street. So are the ten passengers on a metro train when a predator sets upon an innocent.

We can ask ourselves that question again. We can ask it and attempt to answer with examples from the martial way's significant history, or the hallmarks of its traditions, or the extensive beliefs that the antiquity of its thought communicates to us today in its myriad cultural forms. Or we can accede to its simple, undeniable answer and the resolve it compels us to accept.

Why train?

My God, how can we not?

NOTES

1. Petula Dvorak, "Passengers Watched Killing on Metro Car. Should They Have Intervened?" *The Washington Post*, July 9, 2015, accessed September 25, 2017, www.highbeam.com/doc/1P2-38500002.html?refid=easy_hf.

Introduction: The Martial Is Moral

Know Your Ought

When scientists looked to record data on the stimulation of a frog, they used a bell to startle it into jumping. They rang the bell, recorded how far the frog jumped, and then cut off one of its appendages. This ringing and snipping continued until the frog was but a stump. And when they rang the bell for what would be the last time, and Stumpy did not jump, their conclusion was this: when all of a frog's appendages are removed, it loses its hearing.

This story was told to my father in his first year at dental school, and its point is simple: do not disregard the obvious. That's essentially what this whole book is about: rediscovering and clarifying what is, or rather what should be, self-evident truth. Bear in mind, this is not the stuff we all agree on—nobody really agrees on everything anyway— but rather that which we cannot deny.

Imagine training the chest-compression and breathing techniques of CPR but divorced from their purpose of saving lives. Without their purpose, why learn them? What's the point of the skill if we're training ourselves to be incapable of recognizing when it ought to be applied?

In fact, without that "ought," that sense of obligation, what makes it at all necessary?

Some years ago I traveled to the West Coast for training at a weekend event. During one of the segments, I was called to the front to physically defend a fellow who was to be attacked. Now, I was a highly adept martial artist who'd been training since I was a kid, and I'd even lived in Japan for several years, getting my butt kicked by the very best teachers of my art. I was little concerned about defending anybody from anybody because I knew something the attacker did not: I was about to attack the hell out of him.

The moment my protectee was threatened, I leaped into action with more than twenty years of expertise to thwart the assault. I remember feeling pretty satisfied as I loomed over the aggressor, now facedown in the dirt and dust, and twisted him into an airtight submission. I was proud of myself—I'd been called out before a crowd of my peers, so my aim was to impress, and I was pretty sure I had. I remember that moment as well as I remember the next: turning to confirm the safety of my protectee, only I couldn't find him. He'd been silently nabbed by an unknown second attacker. Cue the laugh track for this fool.

A teacher, mentor, and friend, Jack Hoban, arranged the fiasco. He had nothing against me; he was simply taking advantage of the chance to teach a larger lesson. And I have never forgotten that lesson. It laid bare the one thing no professional ever wants to admit he possesses: a weakness he wasn't even aware he had. My confidence to serve up skill lacked the one thing truly necessary for right action: clarity of what I *ought* to do. My job, my role, in that moment was not about attacking an attacker. It was about defending someone, about safeguarding his life. *It was about being a protector.*

After all my years of training and experience, you might think I should have already known this, that it would be second nature, a given. It was not. And it is not for many other professionals. In that crucial moment, I was convinced I was doing the right thing, but I was wrong. I was confused. And I failed. Instead of being a protector, I behaved like a thug.

No one trains martial arts to get worse at martial arts. No one trains to gain less understanding and ability. Everyone trains to get better, gain comprehension, and enlighten themselves. Even weirdos dressed as Power Rangers who flood the net with claims of secret training from Master Cucamonga believe this through the fog of their own self-importance. In fact, it is this unanimous motivation to gain proficiency that's translated into the variety of reasons folks train in martial arts. But real proficiency is contingent on a central truth: it must protect and defend a clear sense of obligation. It must know its ought.

In his seminal work, *The Twenty Guiding Principles of Karate*, the founder of modern karate, Gichin Funakoshi, recounts the story of a famous feudal-age sword master. A high-level student of Tsukahara Bokuden with "extraordinary technical skill" passed by a skittish horse, which kicked at him. The student "deftly turned his body to avoid the kick and escaped injury." Townsfolk were so impressed, they immediately related the story to Bokuden himself, who reportedly said, "I've misjudged him," and promptly expelled the student.

Mystified by his reasoning, folks plotted to force Bokuden to react to the same circumstances. They placed "an exceedingly ill-tempered horse" on a road they knew he used, then secretly waited. When the old man finally came round, they were surprised to see him give the horse a wide berth and pass without incident. Once the townspeople confessed their ruse, the sword master said this: "A person with a mental attitude that allows him to walk carelessly by a horse without considering that it may rear up is a lost cause no matter how much he may study technique. I thought he was a person of better judgment, but I was mistaken."[1]

Funakoshi highlights this story to introduce the principle of "mentality over technique," writing "mentality" as *shinjutsu*, describing acute mindfulness with ethical connotations. Losing our mentality, or, worse, being willfully ignorant of it, can be life threatening, as it represents a personal duty. Bokuden dismissed his student for the plainest of reasons: *he had lost touch with the duties he was obligated to uphold to himself. And if he had failed himself, what use was he to anyone else in need?*

This clarity of obligation is by far the most important point of martial undertaking because it places every lesson in context—protecting the self grants the confidence and accountability to protect others. People concoct all kinds of reasons to study the martial way, but track those reasons far enough, and they invariably travel full circle to this originating alpha point because of a shared experience: *the martial way was not invented; it was discovered.*

Universal instincts from deep within the human condition compelled early adherents toward a shared sense of purpose: to survive human conflict. Thus, at different times, in different places, by different people, in different ways around the world, the martial way was realized and refined into the plurality of means and methods we know today. More than simply traditions of culture or libraries of fighting techniques, they are creeds. Codified systems imbued with values, morals, ethics, and virtues—a code of what we feel, what we think, what we do, and what we aspire to do—all calibrated to a particular end, what I call the *protector ethic.*

The Protector Ethic

Take this true story of a young man who went to the aid of a young woman—she was being beaten. This fellow tried to thwart the attack by attacking her attacker. But, unbeknownst to our hero, the aggressor's friends were not far behind, and when they came on their comrade receiving a knuckle sandwich, they served up several of their own. Whatever happened to the girl is anyone's guess.

Were our hero's actions ethical? Did he do the right thing?

He saw the violence and knew it was wrong. This young lady did not deserve to be beaten by a cretin. In his gut, he knew this to be immoral and acted. Our hero, a trained martial artist, gained tactical advantage and took the bully out. Now, had the violence stopped at that point, perhaps he could've tipped his hat and walked into the sunset. But the question remains: Did his tactical action provide him with the best option to stop the violence and prevent more?

Some will say yes, based on his *intention* to do right. But intending is not the same as doing. Knowing the right is not enough—doing the right is what counts. Then perhaps by merit of the *outcome*? Still not enough. The outcome could have been born of pure luck, like a rum-fueled dance-like-nobody's-watching stumble accidentally knocking the attacker out—hardly an ethical act, even when the outcome goes his way. But the outcome didn't go his way, and our hero was lucky he won only some nasty bruises, in spite of doing a noble, dumb thing that could have resulted in croaking at the hands of angry drunks.

The world is a brutal place, and there will always be cases in which good folks have no choice but to attack an attacker, even at great risk to themselves or others. But this doesn't mean it should be our first choice. In fact, if your default setting in regular training is "stomping mudholes in chests" or worse, slitting throats like a commando but you are not a commando, you are priming yourself to go off road, even off map, to cause greater conflict and violence. "Kill 'em all and let Gary sort 'em out" is an awful way for Gary to live in the real world, where some of that indiscriminate aggression will rub off on him and people he cares about.

We can be tactical without being ethical. It's easy, really—far easier than being both, for sure. Even though our hero had been tactical—he approached and ambushed unseen from the rear—he had not acted on the ethical first. If he had, he would have given himself the best opportunity for the outcome he was initially compelled to effect.

Let's remember why he intervened to begin with. It wasn't to deliver justice to the villain and tie him up with a note for the cops. He did it to protect a young woman who could not protect herself. Why, then, did he choose a tactic that endeavored the former and neglected the latter? Bear in mind, once the aggressor's friends attacked our hero, it created a new issue: now he needed defending. And the young woman was left in the very same predicament our hero found her in to begin with—at the mercy of those who meant her harm. *He had lost touch with the duties he was obligated to uphold to himself. And if he had failed himself, what use was he to anyone else in need?*

By unnecessarily attacking the attacker, the hero placed himself, the girl, and even his attackers in potentially deadly harm. Yes, even his attackers: had the hero or someone else been carrying a concealed weapon, such as a firearm, it might have turned into a turkey shoot with no turkeys.

What ought the hero have done?

He should have placed himself between the young woman and her abuser and separated them. This ethical action is the best tactical action, as it protects everyone:

- By standing up for the girl, he becomes a guardian to protect her from further violence.
- By not immediately attacking the attacker, our hero protects himself because the attacker isn't forced into a fight. Fighting becomes a choice the attacker has to make.
- It also protects the attacker from harm by the hero, as well as harm he may incur on himself as a result of his own poor behavior, even if he doesn't realize it.

Our hero should have acted as a protector of self and others, including, if possible, the enemy. This outlines the protector ethic, with the "if possible" as the balance, since we must engage from a sober understanding of our ability under given conditions—we can only do what we are confident we are capable of doing. Protecting our enemy is definitely the most difficult and dangerous thing we can do. It doesn't just speak to our willingness to do it; it also speaks to our martial capability and maturity because there is no higher skill than to subdue an aggressor without killing him.

Operating from the perspective that less is definitely more, when engaging in violence we should employ the least deadly tactic (until more lethal ones are required), in order to conform with the protector ethic. We should take the application of martial tactics as seriously as any mortal threat posed against us. The human body is a complex, if sometimes frail, vessel that can malfunction just as often as it can perform wondrous feats. How an opponent will react in response to grave techniques is often an educated guess. Every year there are an alarming number of scuffles that turn deadly—one-punch knockouts that end up homicides, and this often between untrained people. And let's face it: any physical action we perform may land us in court, since in this polite society, litigiousness is a culling sword, even when folks follow the law and do everything right.

Balancing the ethical-tactical continuum is the best way to increase our ability because it's when we can (or cannot) ethically protect everyone and resolve conflict that tactics become vividly clear. The tactical itself, on its own, is devoid of meaning without orientation—a sword-cutting technique is simply that, a procedure to cut with a sword. The technique gains priority and consequence only when used in fulfilling our protector ethic, which is always moral-physical.

A Moral-Physical Philosophy

Some believe the ethical and tactical are mutually exclusive, even incompatible. The tactical is about survival, they'll say—"Kill or be killed." The ethical is for Sunday school or philosophers, who rarely, if ever, get punched in the face. But this is hardly true—I get punched all the time.

Anytime someone decides to begin martial training, the decision itself is of an ethical nature. Take the three most basic questions anyone who trains must answer:

What am I going to learn?
How am I going to learn it?
Whom am I going to learn from?

These considerations only gain in importance because they do not just inhabit teaching lives; they haunt them:

What am I going to teach?
How am I going to teach it?
Whom am I going to teach?

We answer these questions regardless of our awareness or ignorance of them because choosing to train in martial arts is our vote for the "what, how, and whom." These questions further call for direction, not just for knowledge of techniques but also for the manner of their use. Manners relate to a person's qualities, and qualities relate to character. "Manners are of more importance than laws," the philosopher Edmund Burke wrote. "Manners are what vex or soothe, corrupt or purify, exalt or debase, barbarize or refine us, by a constant, steady, uniform, insensible operation, like that of the air we breathe in."[2] No one can engage the martial without being subjected to the modification of character.

Training does not automatically moralize us just because we do it. It only grants us the opportunity, provided we affix training to its virtuous, life-protecting design. Unless students are faced with the inherent duties of the protector ethic, training is nothing but selfish endeavor. One that can become incomprehensible if we purposely obscure its path due to our own penchant for amusement, or, worse, outright refusal to follow the path where it's taking us. The biggest concern anyone should have with training is the obsession with technical information—techniques—which is symptomatic of the excessive focus on the self and the continual satisfaction of the ego. Perhaps you've heard martial arts destroys the ego, but this is silly. People need a healthy ego to thrive. Training functions as a temper, and it does so by balancing our needs and wants with humility stemming from our duties to self and others.

When training gets selfish, it can grow dark and twisted, a place where everyone is a potential enemy, including people we care about. Instead of becoming that happier, healthier, brighter light to the world that others look to for strength and guidance, we dim, obscured by shadows of our own making. And it's only in this darkness that the bloodline of the martial way is misidentified as mere "killing arts." This has the effect of diminishing it, severing the link between tactical strategies and their original, life-protecting principles. The account departs from any sense of responsibility and appeals, perhaps unwittingly, to a base appetite for "might makes right," a self-satisfaction that degrades training as amoral, neither ethical nor unethical. If it's neither right nor wrong, it's just a cold, hard tool that makes it easy to kill.

Now, do not misunderstand me. The knowledge and material ability to kill an enemy hold an immeasurably important place—sacred, even— in martial means and ways. In many respects, maturity in the martial way is paradoxical, as in "learning to die in order to live" or "killing to protect life." These notions are intrinsic to advanced studies, but because they are not simple to comprehend, let alone physically embody, they are easily misunderstood. And the easiest to misinterpret is the martial as merely mortal.

The fate of the feudal and ancient world was indiscriminate death. People died young, sick, and infirm, as they were plagued by plagues, starved, hunted, and massacred between tribes and clans. History's brutality is legendary. It was the martial way that tipped the balance to protect and sustain life. Is there any question as to why the warrior class would ascend to the preeminent cultural position throughout antiquity? It wasn't because the warrior was renowned for his death dealing, but his life protecting. Death was commonplace. Life was special.

If the guiding value of the martial way is only the killing of the enemy, then how do we explain the fact that these ancient arts retain the tactical calculations in order *to live* through battling an enemy, even though killing may be necessary? It is always far easier to kill and train to kill when one's life is sacrificial to that goal. Terrorism's use of the suicide bomb is first and foremost for killing because its aim places it above even the life of the bomber. But the martial way actually coheres to human nature's life-preserving instincts—even a survival martial art is qualified by the value-of-life notion, survival.

When we depict and participate willingly in a so-called killing art, we revoke training's ethical standard. And even if we acknowledge the standard, if we don't train, articulate, and rely on it, we leave it to the misinformed and uninitiated to use its absence against us in a court of public opinion. And, worse, perhaps one dark day in an actual court, where the fearful among us will state the argument for its abolition. It wouldn't be the first time.

The way of the martial is moral. Whenever we use it, train in it, or teach it to others, we deal with the ethical, the moral in action. And the protector ethic is the outstanding bond, the summit of its endeavor, *why* it all matters in the first place. Believe it or don't—*the martial way is ruled from within the realm of ethics.*

Every physical technique and tactic, every philosophical and strategic conjugation of use, is contingent on this singular point. It is the self-evident, undeniable way of the martial way.

On Ethics

Ethics is as complicated as martial arts, which is to say, as complex as we wish to make it. There are plenty of rabbit holes down which practitioners can fall, but at its most basic, ethics deals with primarily three sets of issues:

- Good and bad, which concerns the values we value
- Right and wrong, which involves how we reason and judge to uphold our values
- Decisions and actions we take to protect and preserve those aspects

Martial ethics deals with how we answer threats and violence when values contradict. Understanding how and why values come into opposition is central to defusing that conflict. Human values are only ever *objective*—shared by everyone, such as necessities for sustenance—or *subjective*—relative, shared only by some, such as those dictated by culture or creed. Nutrition is an objective value because if we don't get it, we die. But your favorite football team is your subjective, arbitrary choice. Objectivity trumps subjectivity, always and every time. If it's up to us to arbitrate between them, not only must we know good from bad, right from wrong, and how to act on these concerns, we have to first identify the subjectivity causing trouble and activate objectivity to alleviate it.

Applying an objective ethic means seeking the universal because it is just as it sounds: good for all involved. If protectors don't deal in universals, then their thoughts, words, and deeds remain untrustworthy to those who are forced to live by their decisions and actions.

The ethical measure of decisions often comes down to how well they apply to everyone equally. Equality begins with trying to protect everyone in conflict—victims and perpetrators—basing decisions and actions on changing circumstances or context. If protectors do not treat everyone equally, decisions will become suspect, as will the protectors themselves, and it will foment more conflict.

Perhaps more important, without universals, protectors risk having their own thoughts, words, and deeds mutate and work against them. Doing the right thing means knowing how to discover what that right thing is. But if that's done through disrespect, then protecting actually becomes bullying. This can cause confusion, frustration, and even physical sickness to those involved. Protectors need clarity to trust their decision making, since they're the ones who must ultimately live with the decisions they may be forced to make.

In seeking the universal, we have to ask questions like, What is good? and, before this, What is valuable? And we must clarify what it means to value at all. These are the starter questions of ethics, and it's good training to provide answers here, even if they're difficult or confusing at first.

Can we know if any of our answers will approach truth? Moral truth? Unfortunately, much of the world will inform us this is irrelevant. It will say humans operate by "moral relativism," meaning we cannot know with certainty the actuality of rightness, goodness, or moral values, as these are mere projections of culture and experiences distinct to us. As such, they are mere opinions, as particular as any partisan's. Perhaps you stand with those folks and think that terms like *objective*, *universal*, and *absolute* cannot possibly pertain to moral thinking, and even less attain truth, in a world with infinite shades of gray.

Let's sidestep the fact that condemning the possibility of objective, absolute statements of moral truth is in itself an objective, absolute statement of moral truth. Moral relativism is a colloquialism of a popular theory, as we'll learn later, that people pick up and swing around as easily as a child's plastic bat. When conceived as an "ethical" method, it provides tacit cover to legitimize not doing the right thing when the right thing needs to be done. Worse, it insists there can be no knowing the right thing.

Wrong.

At one of the many speeches G. K. Chesterton, the English writer and Catholic apologist, gave during his time, a reporter asked which book, if he could have any single book, he would want if stranded on a desert island. Such a learned and literary fellow must have some deep insight. Would he choose the King James Bible or a volume of Shakespeare? Nope. *Thomas' Guide to Practical Shipbuilding*.

There's a standard in his answer, one that cannot be unseated even by academics who make careers, some very successful, out of studying precisely which book is the best book to be stranded on a desert island with. These folks are outsmarting themselves—any other book is simply a matter of taste. Only Chesterton's answer reminds us there is a whole world to see, one wholly worth seeing if only we could get the hell off that sandbar.

This is the essential difference between the relative and the universal, the subjective and the objective, the arbitrary and the absolute. And it outlines the real challenge in the study of ethics, especially in the study of martial ethics: to discern the truth of the good and then protect and defend it. If we're willing to fight, or protect others from harm, or hurt, maim, or kill those who might do the harming, we had better be able to explain not only the good reasons, but the *just* reasons we fought for and defended others. We had better be able to clarify *why*.

In seeking the universal, what is good for everyone, we first need some context for what it is we're searching for, thus the question, *what is the nature of human nature?* Is it a book to be read or a book to be written? Is it revealed to us, something we discover and recognize as an answer to what it means to be human? Or is our human nature whatever we conclude is worthwhile through reason and experience?

If our nature is due to reasoned knowledge, acquired through experience, then human nature is a book to be written and ought to be organized as good experiences deemed worthy enough for habituating. Much of Greek philosophy centered on the concept of defining this "good life," *eudaimonia*. Greek thought is really, really old, so this is by no means new.

But here's an older idea.

What is it that deems worthy any collection of experiences, habits, or traits concerning the good in the first place? What is it that provides the justification for their inclusion? Is it simply the fact that we think they are worthy? We all take a vote and agree they are? Remember, this book is not about what we agree on. We're looking instead for what is undeniable.

Could there be an ardent standard by which our "good" ideas could be judged? Perhaps one that is more important and of greater value than fickle human opinion? Could there be a concept that is so cherished that even the good itself could be appraised against it to determine if it is in fact "good"?

There is.

What More than This?

In graduate school, I wrote a paper in which I made the case that certain human values—truth telling, prohibition on murder, and valuation of the young—are nonnegotiable. This means they require both our protection and profound respect.

Truth telling protects the functioning of an interconnected society that relies on accuracy in measurements and communications. Imagine if ground control lied to airlines about the weather or engineers fabricated dimensions in the construction of bridges and buildings. Chaos would ensue since we could never be sure if we were being told the truth. Every individual has an inalienable right to their existence, and the prohibition on murder embraces this right as the foundation of societal laws and mores. If the unborn, babies, and children were not protected and instead were killed, they could not grow up to replace older and dying members of society. And if wholesale violation of all these values were to occur in some anarchic scenario, it would jeopardize the collapse of any society.

These three values are not merely good ideas; they are crucial, fundamental, and necessary to human existence and its flourishing. Not only does this make their inclusion in the pantheon of cherished human values obvious, but it also designates them as something special: *moral*. How we understand what is moral has everything to do with how we value. *And how we value has everything to do with how we value life.*

Whenever we discuss the load-bearing walls of ethics, we wind up reaching for this concept called *normativity*. A "normative source" is like the Ark of the Covenant, the Sankara Stones, the Holy Grail, and that silly crystal skull all rolled into one fortune-and-glory McGuffin of moral philosophy. Think of it as a quantum or string theory that moors our disparate emotions, mindful concerns, and physicality to a single dock. It provides an explanation for why we feel, think, and do the way we feel, think, and do. This isn't simply defining what drives the car but rather unraveling the theory of combustion that necessitates the form of the engine, which in turn designates the design of the car, and even shapes the manner of its use.

Only a value for life provides the set of inclinations humans have to naturally protect, defend, and sustain it. Our cells fight off viruses; our immune systems create tolerances to bacteria; our brains process fear and purpose adrenaline, driving neural instincts to concentrate blood and raise our heart rates to help us defend ourselves or flee from an attack; and our consciousness teams with our proprioception to navigate a world that can harm us. From our cellular structure to our spiritual consciousness, even to the surprising number of failed suicides—most—we humans are designed to be life-sustaining creatures.

The value of life is the nature of our human nature, the book that is read, and thus revealed to us, and is the wellspring for our sense of normative obligation, one that recognizes self-evident behaviors that support our care and protection.

It's no mistake that within the annals of martial history, the highest order of mastery has always been to undo the enemy while sparing his life, if at all possible. And within the philosophic realm, the value of life is the source of justification for our visceral instincts of obligation to care for ourselves and others. What other earthly validation exists to make sacred our highest conception of values, in the form of morals, ethics, justice, and rights? What good would any of these notions be if they were twisted to violate and ravage, operating in contradiction to the existence of human "being"?

If you're not convinced that the power of morals, ethics, justice, and rights is due to the value we place on life, then ask yourself this: Why do these things matter anyway? What is it that makes them valuable in the first place? Is it simply because we agree they are? Do they only matter as much as the prevailing opinion held by those who vote for them at the time? A 51 percent rule is a dangerous precept for discovering moral clarity considering that collective human agreement is as foolproof as picking up a bucket while you are in it.

There is an intrinsic quality that makes these metaphysical concepts valuable, even if the majority of us agreed they were not of value. What invigorates them must be the value of life because that is what they aim to protect and defend. If the dignity of human being were somehow of no importance to our experience, then these concepts would not exist because they would not have mattered enough to be articulated over the course of history. You can't have ideals like morals, ethics, justice, and rights if there is nothing about life ideally worth protecting.

And just why do we value life? What is it that compels us to value our lives and judge everything else by its sustainable accord? Here's my answer after years of research, study, teaching, and contemplation: *we don't know; we just know.*

Did God put it there? Maybe. Is it evolutionary residue? Perhaps. The fact that humans value life is an inescapable truth of the natural world. It shares the stage with other natural truths, such as the four fundamental forces of physics, or the elements that make up the primary constituents of matter.

If we can fulfill the protector ethic—protecting ourselves, those around us, and even our enemy, if at all possible—we will have realized the essence, the root, the core of every core value that has ever shaped the martial way. In fact, we cannot formulate any martial value, including self-confidence, honor, integrity, loyalty, humility, discipline, or inner peace, without respect for the value of life that makes any of them a worthy conception to begin with.

Thus, in taking any martial action for the purposes of defense, what more is there to do than aspire toward the protector ethic? Seriously, I'm asking.

What else ought we try to do? Reduce property damage?

Look Death in the Face

The architect of James Bond, Ian Fleming, drew inspiration from the seventeenth-century Japanese poet Matsuo Basho when he wrote the following iconic words:

> You only live twice:
> Once when you are born
> And once when you look death in the face.[3]

Purposeless death is always an unmitigated tragedy because it thieves from the living. At its least, it's an object lesson that the deceased can never recover and profit from because it denies any chance at renewal, forgoes any do-over, and disallows any potential "rebirth."

Obviously, we live once we realize we are alive. But we also face living once we recognize that we will one day die. This sense of impermanence is an existential crisis we're forced to reconcile throughout our lives by managing our health, our lifestyle, and how the world treats us. To say the crisis does not exist or doesn't impact us is to cast oneself as fool or fraud. Everyone wants a second chance because we are only authentic once we realize it will all end and then play by those rules—the life-preserving ones we want to be judged by and respected for upholding. The same is true for the martial way. It is only authentic once we recognize, train, live, and act on it in ways that correspond to the moral instincts of our humanity.

I have a saying: good people who want to be better people get trained. One of the best ways to become someone who can do more for oneself and others is to train to be more martially able, because

there is no better metric for one's improvement than the ability to miti-
gate both inward and outward conflict.

This is why every individual ought to endure martial training for
some period, if only to reveal the profound ability its skills and philosophy have to empower our sense of self-worth. The protector ethic,
to stand up and defend ourselves and others who might not or cannot
defend themselves, is a habit-formed behavior. Carrying out this ethic
is the heart of any martial art.

Knowing we should do this, and knowing how to accomplish it, is
the difference between accruing mere skill for reenactment and cul-
tivating life-protecting habits. Should we learn the movements of
CPR but devoid of their purpose? A sharper understanding of what
is valuable affords acute mindfulness of what is moral—what we know
we ought to protect. It provides recognition of and clarity regarding
our obligations, and training becomes the direct action of our ethic.

But when we, as this time's undaunted defenders, neoteric teachers,
and persevering guardians of this path, supplant this truth, we get confused: *rather than training techniques to protect and defend life, we
train a life to protect and defend techniques.*

If we are to do right by those in conflict, including ourselves, we
must know that which unlocks the universal. We must apprentice in
honor, integrity, vigilance, and rectitude as the keys to steadfast warriorship. This is nothing less than recognizing the reciprocity of natural justice, instilling temperance in our reasoning, and exhibiting
prudence in our judgment, so we can, above all, have the courage to
act. These cardinal virtues, at least as old as the Greek Stoics, make for
the best map to the protector ethic because if we define ethics as moral
values in action, then martial ethics are moral *protector* values in
action.

To pass on real knowledge and deliver it as wisdom, to teach the
tactical and perceive the ethical, to be exposed to our naturally bind-
ing obligations and by them hold fidelity to their truth so that the next

generation might protect and defend themselves and their families—
I'd argue that's nothing short of God's work.

If we are to fulfill this role, we must hold firm to this certainty: the
martial way only lives once we treat it as something that can die.

NOTES

1. Gichin Funakoshi and Genwa Nakasone, *The Twenty Guiding Principles of Karate* (Tokyo: Kodansha International, 2008), 39.
2. Edmund Burke, *The Works of the Right Honorable Edmund Burke*, rev. ed., vol. 5 (Boston: Little, Brown, 1866), 5:310.
3. Ian Fleming, *You Only Live Twice* (New York: Penguin, 2003), 109.

1

To Value: Justice as Honor

A Genuine Fake

The video is grainy. A blotchy corner timestamp says December 19, 2003, 10:46 a.m. A barren table and a single chair sit against the wall opposite the camera, crowding a small police interrogation room. A scruffy-haired, bearded man is led in by a detective and seated. He's agitated, exposed. In the din of our Verbal Judo classroom, Dr. George "Doc" Thompson points to the projection screen, "This guy just shot a cop." Everyone watching is silently queasy. We oughta be. We're about to witness something awful.

The scruffy man is Ricardo Alfonso Cerna, a Guatemalan immigrant to the United States, and he knows something his captors do not: his latest act of violence will be his third strike in the criminal justice system and assures he'll go to prison for life.

Cerna had just been pulled over by Sheriff's Deputy Michael Parham for a traffic infraction when he decided a high-speed chase would be more exciting. He took off in his vehicle, and when he crashed it, he burst from the wreck in a Butch and Sundance blaze, firing six shots at the deputy, striking him twice in the abdomen. Parham survived.

Several departments then teamed together to run Cerna down and arrest him. In the video, he sits at the San Bernardino sheriff's office in Muscoy, California. The detective who led him in hands him a bottle of water with a good-natured "Here you go, *señor*." The politeness is hard to square with the knowledge that Parham is at this very moment fighting for his life in surgery, a fact the detective must certainly be aware of, but his attitude does not betray. Thompson speaks up: "That just saved his life."

The detective leaves. Cerna opens the bottle, drinks deep, and gives himself a moment. He tugs at his shirt and, like a rabbit from a hat, produces a model 1911 .45-caliber handgun from his waistband. Without hesitation, as if it were a practiced, automatic movement, he presses the muzzle to his temple and blows his brains out.

The blast jolts him stiff. The gun slides from his grip. Blood pours out of him and tattoos the concrete floor like spilled wine. His eyes swell. His nose drips. His body deflates. The detective walks back in. "Aww fuck. Nobody shook him [searched him]." Cerna's head lolls, his body sinking heavily but still in his seat. "Holy fuck." The video darkens.

Even though the San Bernardino police, the county sheriff, and the California Highway Patrol all had a hand in arresting Cerna, no one had properly searched him. Investigators would later confirm that his gun had two bullets left.

Cerna's violence toward an officer might have won him disdain, causing the detectives to vent anger against him. It's possible no one would have thought twice about it if they did. But because the detective's treatment of Cerna exemplified a universal truth—everyone wants to be treated with dignity—he didn't arm Cerna with a motive to kill him.

Several years ago I was invited to complete a forty-hour course in Verbal Judo. If you're unfamiliar with it, look it up. It's known today as TacComm, or Tactical Communication, and its founder, the late Dr. Thompson, started teaching it more than thirty years ago after earning a PhD in English literature, then serving some twenty years in law enforcement, where he refined its techniques. The video was one of many, illustrating that our words can either keep us a step ahead or push us off a cliff.

Thompson, a longtime martial artist himself, described Verbal Judo as a "martial art of the mind," and he was right. Verbal Judo's principles are based on observation of the human condition and designed to take advantage of another's verbal aggression, tip them off balance, and gain control. He spoke about letting go of one's ego, maintaining one's temper, focusing only on another's behavior, letting angry words wisp away. Thompson even said he'd reconciled police tactics with Aristotelian models of rhetorical persuasion and laid it all out in clear form. The secret to it was what he called *tactical courtesy*.

Throughout that weeklong course, there were endless examples of people saving lives using a mind trained in tactical courtesy as a baseline for conduct. This means treating others, including despicable criminals, with the same level of basic courtesy we'd ourselves like under similar conditions. Stories were varied, and many included officers using their words to deescalate situations. One legendary LA gang detective unknowingly saved his own life one night: a bogus 911 call was actually an initiation to assassinate a cop. But when this detective showed up, the gangsters lowered their rifles, explaining some months later that their regard for him—because of the regard he had shown them—stayed their triggers. Thompson himself was called in to negotiate with an unstable father holding a knife to the throat of his three-year-old son. No one wanted bloodshed, but SWAT snipers were already in place and needed but a sign to take a shot, so Thompson combed the man's words for the key to use against him. When finally admitting he did not want to kill his son but he felt he had to—he was possessed by the devil— there it was. Thompson suggested a priest perform an exorcism. It worked. The boy was unharmed and his father taken into custody.

Like any rhetoric, be it the timing of comedy, riposte in debate, or eloquence in speech, tactical courtesy is a practiced skill, rife with

3

techniques and tactics that must be studied under expert practitioners and applied unceasingly. At its best it can deliver a masterstroke when the practitioner is under duress.

But good timing does not make one funny, clever riposte does not ensure one argues from the truer perspective, and stirring speech certainly does not imbue the message with meaning and profundity. Like politeness or civil manners, especially under stressful or taxing conditions, tactical courtesy is a performance, a veneer. Don't get me wrong, compelling another's compliance in lieu of conflict is an excellent skill for any professional.

However, there's a principle here worth embracing because it's the fundamental building block for strategies like tactical courtesy and virtue itself: *genuine respect.*

Respect is rooted in the protector ethic's first steadfast virtue, honor, and within the ancient cardinal virtue, justice. How we respect—value ourselves and others—and how we uphold that respect, honor, has everything to do with how we justify our reasoning, judgments, and, most importantly, actions.

Respect: Owed or Earned?

Is respect earned or freely given? How would you explain the feeling of basic respect, let alone describe its delivery—what does it mean to show respect? And can we stomach giving it to those we might deplore, like an enemy, opponent, or criminal?

In much of the martial way, the beginning and end of training are marked by respect, or *Rei*. We bow upon entry to our training space, we treat our teachers with deference, and we protect our training partners, though we may seem to mistreat them through the rigors of training itself. For much of our everyday life, many would agree that showing respect means adhering to the Bible's Golden Rule: "Do unto others as you would have them do unto you" (Matt. 7:12). The concept is simple, as it relies on our own self-worth in balancing treatment of and from others.

But is this arguably self-evident point flawed? One person's standards can differ from another's and so may be perceived as offensive by another. This would mean the Golden Rule isn't so shiny because to treat others in a way that they consider offensive would be to treat them disrespectfully. This has led to calls to revise the Golden Rule into: "Treat others the way *they* wish to be treated."

However, this is the same issue in reverse—the behavior of others might be considered offensive by you. Allowing our actions to be governed by the quirky tastes of another person's culture or creed, especially if those ways are unknown to us and out of context, is counterproductive at the least. Imagine police officers treating the public, suspects, and criminals by the variable cultural standards *they* wish to be treated by. Deference to this subjectivity would engage police in endless study of cross-cultural and sociological trends, with the result that police would "respect" some people differently from other people under similar circumstances, turning law enforcement into awful enforcement.

Does Kant hold the answer? Immanuel Kant was an eighteenth-century German philosopher who channeled the Golden Rule into his own maxim stating we should always treat others as "ends" in themselves and never merely as "means" to our own ends. In his *Groundwork for the Metaphysics of Morals*, he reinforced his ideas with his "categorical imperative": "Act only according to that maxim whereby you can, at the same time, will that it should become a universal law."[1] That's a fancy way of saying, do only that which you would be willing to have everyone else do to everyone—including you—all the time.

But even Kant's meticulous phrasing requires qualification, since his formulation could be applied to almost anything, and, in fact, it was sometimes interpreted to that end, such as when the Nazis used Kant to justify their most heinous actions. Kant was named as a forefather of the ideals of Nazis from Adolf Hitler to Adolf Eichmann, chief logistician of the Holocaust. Eichmann, kidnapped in Argentina by the Israeli Mossad and extradited back to Israel, famously argued at his trial in 1961 that he attempted to live his life by Kant's categorical imperative, saying, "'True to the law, obedient, a proper personal life, not to come into conflict with the law.' This, I would say, was the categorical imperative for a small man's domestic use." In other words, I was only following orders when I enabled a precision plan to boxcar Jews for extermination in death camps. Now, philosophical Kantians are, of course, dismissive here, and they are wont to say, "The Nazis didn't get Kant right." Of course they didn't get him *right*. But tell that to the Nazis.

Getting it right is an enduring problem when seeking prescribed formal guidance, whether it's from Socrates or Bruce Lee, because throughout the ages, well-meaning sentiments have fallen casualty to misinterpretation and outright misuse in disciplines ranging from philosophy to theology. Even the Bible's Ten Commandments, some of world's oldest moral directives, have created confusion. "Thou shalt not kill" has been ridiculed, as any plain reading can prompt one to question the butchery of animals and discount self-defense and just war. But the misunderstanding stems from translation—the original Hebrew actually said, "Thou shalt not murder." The fact is that the human condition too often grinds both the intellectually complex and sublime into a digestible paste, allowing us to gorge all the better on the feeling of moral superiority, a permanent human failing.

What's misunderstood in criticism of the Golden Rule is simply this: it is not formalized but *empirical* by nature, meaning it requires observation and experience rather than mere reliance on theory, logic, or platitude. To use it correctly—that is, respectfully—we're obliged to seek further content, such as given conditions dictating our behavior and manners, and better understand the context of use, such as why we are engaged with someone to begin with, before we make it a sound maxim. With this combination of the moral context and physical conditions, we can create a behavioral ideal for everyday ethics and true up moral-physical endeavor, be it religion, secular theory, or martial art.

An important way to achieve this is to discard the misguided notion that respect should be "earned." Earning respect is not about respect at all, per se, and, frankly, not what people actually mean when they speak of it.

We earn a personal sense of trust, integrity, and admiration when we prove ourselves competent in thought, word, or deed. Call it what you will—capability, aptitude, experience, or know-how—fraternalism occurs whenever truth and the adversity of its discovery are revealed and shared, be it physically or metaphysically. Often enough, the idea of earning respect is simply an excuse to treat others unequally or unfairly unless or until they've "measured up" in a way sometimes unknown or improbable for them. Daily respect toward others does not and should not have a requirement to be earned, since it has little to do with the receiver and everything to do with its giver.

The word *respect* comes from the Latin *respectus*, "regard, a looking at," and, literally, "an act of looking back (or often) at one." We "pay respects" to people because of their authority or status, even if we deplore them. "Last respects" are offered at a funeral in regard to the life lived by the individual, no matter how good a life led. A moment of silence is given "in respect"—in deference—to those who lost their lives, whether you knew them or not. Respect as a basic concept and a behavioral ideal is bought and paid for by our very lives—we need not know others intimately or admire their abilities to acknowledge them with "respect/s." Much as love is given freely, often for unexplainable reasons and regardless of the individual's personal failings, respect is bestowed on others as a service toward the dignity of their life.

To expect everyone we encounter to "measure up" to our own personal truths, based on our culture, creed, politics, profession, race, religion, identity, values, or beliefs, is tantamount to a prejudicial test—the satisfaction of a personal bias before acknowledging that a life has any worth. This is no different from the so-called fix for the Golden Rule,

"Treat others the way *they* wish to be treated." Can you live up to everyone else's personal biases? No, of course not—no one can, nor should they be expected to. Why do people become angry and frustrated when simple respect is withheld from them? Because when not "paid respects" it implies their lives have nothing worth paying for—no value—unless they measure up to an arbitrary and subjective vision—a malicious attitude that only stokes conflict.

Thus, freely conferring our own personal sense of dignity, our "self-respect," on the lives of others is an overtly ethical action, since it's to risk ourselves for another in the face of clear potential conflict. Applying our dignity to the lives of others *defends us* because it actively *protects others*—the very essence of the Golden Rule. Genuine respect then, means exposing and risking ourselves to protect others.

The best physical example of the Golden Rule is probably the most powerful technique in the world. It's thousands of years old, spans cultures throughout the globe, and has done more good and probably saved more lives than just about any other technique—*the handshake.*

In his "Begum of Bengal" speech of 1907, Mark Twain called it

> a most moving and pulse-stirring honor—
> the heartfelt grope of the hand,
> and the welcome that does not descend from the pale,
> gray matter of the brain,
> but rushes up with the red blood of the heart.[2]

The handshake is historically known as a display of peace that demonstrates that the participants carry no weapons. According to legend, the handshake is specifically performed with the left hand in West Africa because participants dropped the weapon from the right and the shield from the left, expressing they had no attack and no means of defending one. I can't think of a better way to express respect to another person, as we are conveying and discerning something like reciprocal trust or a sense of equality to the person we're meeting. If you don't believe so, think about offering your hand to someone and having them refuse it. Feel respected?

From a martial point of view, handshaking is capable of changing a single moment: approaching someone with an extended hand and warm smile creates an opportunity to lead them to do the same by means of our intention—an expression of vulnerability. This opportunity creates a shield of protection because any movement outside of reciprocation indicates noncompliance or, worse, danger. This is why the martial way is so valuable. By physically defending against violence, we train to place ourselves at risk in order to prevent it. And this allows for the very best form of conflict resolution: the unrestricted conferring of respect to acknowledge the implicit worth of the other. Not only that, it creates a powerfully strong, tactical advantage. Marine Corps major Michael Samarov had one such revelation during his tour in Iraq:

> Samarov told the story of how a group in his unit rounded a corner one day and came on an Iraqi funeral procession, which, in traditional fashion, featured both gunfire and shouts. What to do in such a case? Draw your weapons in defense? Protect the procession in case there is violence? Disrupt the procession by passing? Such a situation isn't covered in any field manual. Making a split second decision, a young corporal ordered the troops to lower their guns, remove their helmets and bow. The Iraqis, after a pause, broke into applause. It was a brilliant stroke. Samarov said there was never again any problem in that neighborhood. And it was the result of trying to pull the best possible idea out of thin air and hoping it is the right choice. In Iraq, there are a lot of moments like that.[3]

To embrace the protector ethic is nothing less than to embrace the mantle of ethical leadership. This is because protectors make for good leaders, good leaders are ethical, and ethical leaders alleviate conflict by hazarding the very kind of personal confrontations that cause many to seek their protection in the first place.

Moral concerns can be discovered and idealized, but they must, in the end, be turned into words and deeds. It's our actions, our treatment of others under the auspices of context and conditions, that ultimately make any physical philosophy worthy of study. Fighting the good fight must always partner with writing the good write because it is simply too easy to dismiss ideology alone. But everyone is compelled to take seriously those who risk themselves for others—we're simply wired that way.

Just values can lead to just reasons, judgments, and actions—treating oneself and others *justly*—which is a service to ourselves and others that emanates from our basic sense of common humanity: respect for others applied from our own self-respect. The basis for true justice.

Justice or Just-Us?

So let's talk justice. Define it, right now—picture it in your mind and explain it out loud to an imaginary friend. And challenge yourself—do so in the affirmative, by describing what it *is*, rather than what it *is not*. By now, we've been well trained by outrage from media, social and otherwise, on what *injustice* feels like. But unraveling its pure form is not so easy.

The latter cardinal virtues are far simpler: *temperance* as disciplined self-restraint, *prudence* as wisdom in judgment, and *fortitude* as courage of the will. Already our kinship with these is acute, precisely because justice has been defined variably.

Is justice only achievable under the law? Or is there such a thing as personal, *natural* justice? And if there is, can protectors, warriors, and martial artists embrace it as a personal virtue?

When folks appeal to the concept, as in, "No justice, no peace!" or when Dr. Martin Luther King Jr. said, "The arc of the moral universe is long, but it bends toward justice," these are clear pleas to its tradition of moral authority, so any conception must account for it and even resolve how it's established.

Equality and fairness, though often characteristic in its definition, more likely result from its moral condition, but they are not its source material, since they are descriptive of states of being but not the states themselves. In appealing to them, we would further ask, what *makes* for equality and fairness, what are they in reference to, and what is the locus of their meaning? Thus, a fully formed account cannot be chipped from those single blocks.

Note: You may want to reread that last bit, because I'm saying that justice is not reducible to what most folks typically believe it is—equality or fairness. I think it's more than that. Lest we forget, justice is a societal need, concerning macro aspects such as equality, but it's also a personal one, as it's how our values invoke their moral force and justify righteous action.

Then is it righteousness we seek? "Social" justice has become a media darling of the twenty-first century precisely for its steroidal force of righteousness. But like any steroid abuse, it can invariably lead to indiscriminate rage: justice, social justice, and injustice are susceptible to a similar catch—each term can mean whatever its user declares it to mean, even if that's antithetical to cherished notions of the concept.

Without a sense of magnetic north, we navigate by a spinning compass. Consequently, we get lost, a time when justice can mean anything at all and victims of injustice can be anyone for any reason. Standing for the plight of victims is a noble cause, but if each of us acts as if we are relentlessly victimized, it perverts our moral culture from one of dignity, in which the rule of law is sufficient to settle disputes, to one of victimhood, in which dependence on authority is a mania. This appeal to power is not to settle actual disputes but to merge the coercive influence of groupthink with the bullhorn of social media to compel authorities to take action against any and all perceived slights—basically, when people's feelings get hurt. Were it passed as an actual law of the land, it would make it a crime to offend others—the very antithesis of our First Amendment rights to think, speak, worship, and associate as we see fit.

There is a simple truth here: when anyone can be arbitrarily labeled a victim of injustice, no one truly is, as it diminishes actual victims, sentencing them to queue up alongside the perpetually aggrieved. Justice, and especially *social* justice, should embody "justice for all," not "so shall just-us."

What's left unaddressed is the underlying contradiction at the heart of many calls for this brand of "justice": *self-important subjectivity stokes conflict because it undermines universalism.* As we will see, this is the heart of conflict itself.

The integrity of any ethical movement is threatened anytime the concept of the moral is a counterfeit model, be it introduced by commanders or comedians. Actual justice, applied virtuously and impartially, begets the righteousness that aspires toward a moral resolution because it preserves the universal values for all involved, not just the few in conflict. When president Abraham Lincoln signed the Emancipation Proclamation, legally freeing slaves held in the Confederate states at the height of America's Civil War, it was a long overdue act of righteous justice precisely because it reaffirmed the dignity of their lives—and of life itself—overruling any slave's institutionalized dehumanizing station, one that had for generations been societally established as moral and just. Recognition of worth of the innocents among us resolves any question of worth for all of us. In this way, true justice stands in direct opposition to subjectivity and its claims to morality, which only drain justice of its force of authenticity.

The voracious nature of the human need for morality, equality, and righteousness, exposed by our miserable misfires at them, doubles down on the importance for warriors and anyone who deals with conflict, to know natural justice as a virtue, so as to best understand the essence of the moral-physical philosophies that both guide and bind us.

Perhaps now, defining justice entirely by a single word or phrase or movement seems artificial and incomplete because it is.

The Way of Justice

Justice comprises instinct, reason, and obligation, and it results in an insensible *method* by which we vindicate the authenticity of truth and thereby substantiate moral authority.

There are two principles closely connected to the conception of justice: don't lie and don't steal. These moral imperatives are older than their appearance in the Bible, having been handed down through generations, always in accord with any serious theology and philosophy. They would eventually find themselves residing in the precedents of common law, the law of the feudal world, only to be preserved as the basis for positive laws regarding contracts, criminality, and tort, or civil liability.

But why are these two notions perpetually cast as exponents of justice? What is it about truth telling and deference to the property of others that speaks to us through the ages? Much like the Golden Rule, truth telling and prohibitions on stealing are formulations of just behavior that are reflective and empirical—they seek reciprocal conduct from others under similar circumstances in intention and action.

Truth telling—though I would say "truth keeping," as in adherence to immutable standards—is necessary for the health and stability of any cooperation or sustainable relationship, be it economic or emotional. By common law precedents, we know it better as "Do all you say you will do"—the basis for contract law, in which truthfulness is as much a duty to oneself as it is a promise to others. The prohibition on stealing goes even further: "Do not encroach on others or their property," a formulation indicative of "Do no harm" principles, including prohibitions on murder as the "stealing" of the lives of innocents. Thus we return to the idea of reciprocity for mutual benefit as a key component of justice. In fact, the notion is embedded in a phrase we have often heard: justice is blind.

Recall the statue of blind Lady Justice, who stands outside many courts of law as a personification of the Roman goddess Justicia, which in turn is based on Greek and Egyptian goddess mythology. She's memorable by several features: she is a maiden, representing purity; she holds a pair of scales, or balance; she wears a blindfold; and she has a sword, often double edged. Each of these aspects represents a trait in the methodology of justice.

Though the scales have been said to symbolize everything from fair observance under the law to equilibrium between fate and retribution, and even the weighing of a case's strengths and weaknesses, my interpretation differs. Justice is not meant to simply apply under the law. Its conception predates positive law, and, in cases in which the law is actually unjust, it can be appealed to in order to surpass it. Archaeologists believe that the tool known as the scales is probably older than its oldest evidence, some of which was found in the Indus River valley in modern Pakistan and apparently dates to more than two thousand years before the birth of Christ. Artifacts of ancient Egypt include carved stones marked with hieroglyphics for gold, suggesting people used scales to gauge known quantities of value against the unknown to determine a true worth. Rather than simply being used to weigh items, it appears that scales were originally a tool of *appraisal*.

Karl Petruso explains in "Early Weights and Weighing in Egypt and the Indus Valley," "Clearly, some economic advance, such as the sanctioning of the evaluation of a precious material or the assaying of a heavy material in terms of a dear one, prompted the manufacture of this apparatus [scales]. It is commonly assumed that the earliest commodity to be counterbalanced with the stone weights was gold. More important in terms of technology, however, once the principle of weighing was discovered, scales were pressed into use for other commodities and for purposes other than barter, such as, for example, in determining proportions of the components of a metallic alloy."[4]

I submit that the scales held by Justicia are representative of our assessment of absolute truth and any subjective consideration. This harks back to goddess imagery of antiquity that represented both the Egyptian deity Maat and the later Greek goddess Themis, whose name actually translates as "divine law," as ancestors of Justicia and personifications of "divine order" who were known as guardians of law, fairness, custom, balance, morality, harmony, and justice. Papyrus images from the Egyptian Book of the Dead show Maat engaged with the "weighing of the heart," a ritual of the afterlife in which souls were appraised against Maat's "feather of truth" to determine their worth. If the soul was lighter or equal in weight, it was said the person lived a just life.

M. I. Finley explains in *The World of Odysseus*, "There was themis— custom, tradition, folk-ways, mores, whatever we may call it, the enormous power of 'it is (or is not) done.' The world of Odysseus had a highly developed sense of what was fitting and proper." In a footnote he continues, "Themis is untranslatable. A gift of the gods and a mark of civilized existence, sometimes it means right custom, proper procedure, social order, and sometimes merely the will of the gods (as revealed by an omen, for example) with little of the idea of right."[5]

This civilized existence, proper custom, social order, and the divine will all have to do with weighing our own humanness against anything that might challenge its self-evident defining attributes, the most essential of these being that life *is of value in all cases*, no matter who we are or where we come from.

This is a plain truth of the natural world. And the only way to recognize and accept this truth is to "blind" ourselves to it. Justicia's blindfold represents reasoning that impartially detaches from race, creed, and culture; rejecting exclusivity for the human condition; and embracing inclusiveness of the human family. People may talk and act in subhuman ways, but they are no less human than any of us, which is why our judgments of them must be made with the utmost regard for all of us, not just a few.

Justice is the amalgam of identifying natural truth, recognizing it objectively and impartially, and then arming ourselves with that understanding—the double-edged sword—to grant us moral authority, which is both obligatory for ourselves and coercive for others.

Now, though our brains can understand all of this, the way to know justice in its clearest most intense form is when it *feels* right. And that feeling does not come to us by way of the winning argument, newer theory, or specific explanation. No, it comes to us in the best of forms, the kind we are most familiar and comfortable with, and oftentimes makes the most sense: A story.

✳ The Moral as Martial: Honesty

If you're into all this philosophy stuff, great. Not everyone is. Being a martial artist is to be defined, at least in part, by how we engage the physical. To this end, we have to figure out how justice fits into any physical schema. What does it mean to exhibit justice or be "just" in terms of one's martial training? Is there a way we can connect this philosophy to the physical? There is. It's called *honesty*.

In 2014, in the city of Caloocan (pronounced Ca-lo-oh-kan), Philippines, north of Manila, a security guard battled a knife-wielding former employee in a ninety-second murder match. There's video of it online. Watch it if you want nightmares. To see the guard flail for his life, dying in the very office he was manning, is like suffocating from too much fresh air. A large predator stalking us in the wild is bad enough, but a coworker taking advantage of surprise and fear to attack us with a melee weapon can cause even the battle hardened to despair. We can only wish swift justice for the guard's killer, who, as of this writing, is still on the loose. The horror show is a grim reminder of the finality of decisions and actions under the stupefying stresses of violence.

This kind of savagery contributes to ever-present martial debates, in particular, the defense against knives, in which there are two camps in argument, combatists and artists. Think of their difference in terms of driving. Artists provide well-known, traditional techniques to teach drivers good habits. Combatists concentrate on dangerous potentials, like accidents and emergency maneuvers, and focus on "inoculating" participants to aggressively overcome these potentials in kind.

Some combatists make the claim that there is no dependable way to deal effectively with a knife-wielding opponent, and to even try is fool-hardy. It's always better to escape than fight, they say. For evidence they point to training scenarios dubbed "traditional" and "real." They accuse artists of employing outlandish techniques in the safety of the dojo, when they are clearly overwhelmed by a blitz-type attack. To make their point, they screen CCTV recordings of knife attacks, such as that at Caloocan. Combatists warn that artists are fooling themselves, and that by training "unrealistically," they'll only wind up wounded or dead.

There are several challenges to the combatists' claim. If knife defense is irresolvable, then why has it been part of the DNA of martial train-ing for as long as there has been training? How do combatists recon-cile a thousand years of martial refinement in which knives and various bladed weapons and techniques for their defense have held prominent roles in the curriculum of various schools? Why did warriors of old make knife defense a staple in their defensive study? Are we to believe they were faking it? That it's hollow tradition? And why such a focus on the knife? Firearms are far more dangerous, as they can kill at dis-tance and disproportionately deliver lethal results even when wielded by the untrained. And yet, combatists are not making the same argu-ments against gun disarming and their defense.

Three obvious issues also complicate an escape-only policy for any martial concern: context, tactical options, and "viability." Escaping is always a great idea, until it isn't, such as when we can't escape because we must protect someone else. This issue of context is game changing. We may also lose the tactical option to escape if constrained by area or environment, like backed into a corner, again forcing us to fight. And what I call "viability," or life-sustaining use of martial techniques, is challenged whenever escaping actually provides a tactical advantage to an opponent to use the timing of our decisions and actions against us, like running away only to die tired when we're stabbed in the back. Every combatist and artist has a responsibility to recognize the fact that there are going to be certain cases in which we will have to fight no matter what, knife or no knife.

But combatists are onto something. Too many artists are afflicted by a common malady known variously as the inflammation of dojoitus, the code of bullshido, or nonjutsu the ancient and secret art of the nincompoop. These afflictions are all the same: the denial and stripping of honesty from training.

Standards not operative in the real world, existing only in the dojo, can allow artists to shield themselves behind their authority, cultural affectation, or tradition. Under these stipulations, well-meaning cooperative training between willing participants can mutate, even metastasize into reckless enabling to foster confidence in counterfeit skills.

Unfortunately, in martial training this can happen to folks with the best of intentions. It can also lead to wildly irresponsible behavior. In both the East and the West, there is a legendary technique dubbed the "no-touch knockout," in which the practitioner is purportedly able, through fantastical energy or something, to control his attackers without touching them. This type of power has been claimed by a variety of folks, from American teachers to members of Asian organizations that don't amount to much more than cults. In reality, the odds are pretty good these same folks will never use their ability for real-world defense, remaining ever ignorant or dishonest that their skills are nonexistent. That is, unless they discover, most likely under threat, they are reenactors or, worse, outright frauds rather than leaders. It will be a terrifying moment of clarity.

The two ancient principles of justice, don't lie and don't steal, are just as operative in martial training in the service of honesty. First, *we ought not lie to ourselves or others in regard to our skills and ability.* We should take our training seriously and learn from those who take their own training more seriously than we do. The problem for most folks is this: *People want what they want from martial arts—they don't often want what they need.* This is usually due to immaturity and a lack of basic knowledge about what training can actually do. I've met folks who rely on video courses for their training, or equate cosplay and reenactment with bona fide skills, or buy into all manner of wild martial-wizard theory, just to satisfy what they wish they actually knew. It's sad. When I meet folks like this, I usually just give them a handshake and a throaty, "Good luck!" because they're weird and they're probably going to hurt themselves. But it's when those same folks decide they're going to teach others that I get my back up. Lying to yourself is immoral. Acting on it is unethical. But conning others by promising them truths that you don't intimately know yourself borders on sociopathy. At the very least, it makes you an all-around awful person.

The other principle here is don't steal, and it plays directly into how we actually understand our training and accrue ability. The lesson is this: *don't take the truth from others (or yourself) by stealing their chance to reconcile failure.*

If you're training to be a protector, but your actual regimen has as its focus the perfection of movement instead of failing less under stressful conditions, there's a good chance it's simply not going to be as reliable. When training focuses on perfecting itself, or, perfecting technique into performance, this kind of idealization can only occur when the conditions, like resistant partners, are unnaturally controlled—like our "no-touch knockout" friends—to bear no consequences for misuse. But without consequences—read failure—there can be little success.

Success in training is a moment we can inhabit when we reduce our failure-inducing faults—*think "less wrong," not "more right."* Since failure is integral to tracking success, if we don't place ourselves under the conditions of use, and fail, and fail a lot under said conditions, we cannot learn how to fail less by reducing those fault-inducing habits. Fewer faulty habits means less failure, and less failure means a greater chance for success. It may sound a little counterintuitive, but the more you fail, the less you will.

The Hunting Story

The finest example I know to experience and even embed natural justice as a personal virtue is not some scrambled chase down a metaphysical rabbit hole but a simple story—a parable, really, about a real-life search to explain commonsense human equality. It provides guidelines to resolve individual conflict, respect our fellow man, improve cross-cultural relations, and most importantly, reject dehumanization.

Robert L. Humphrey was born in 1923, and his formative years were as a poor child of the Great Depression. He grew up to be a boxcar rambler, a member of Franklin D. Roosevelt's Civilian Conservation Corps, a Golden Gloves boxer, and a merchant marine, and, when he arrived on the island of Iwo Jima in 1945, he was a young Marine Corps rifle platoon lieutenant. At the height of battle, rifle platoon lieutenants had a life expectancy of thirty minutes. Humphrey spent eighteen days on the island before he was wounded.

The Battle of Iwo Jima was war at its vicious and gory pinnacle and every marine has been well schooled in this bloodiest battle of Marine Corps history. It saw more than twenty-two thousand Japanese soldiers shot, blown up, or burned from underground labyrinths and seven thousand marines lose their lives, with countless more wounded. Only 216 Japanese soldiers were taken prisoner at a time when neither side was taking prisoners. On day three of the thirty-six-day fight, six of eight of Humphrey's school friends died within an hour of being brought to the front line.

The island was like a laboratory of horror, a place dominated by a fear so profound it could obscure the better nature of men. Sometimes that resulted in atrocity, like desecration of the dead or abuse of prisoners. But it also inspired magnificence. Feats of valor were too many to count, as men risked their lives for their missions and each other, even when they were sure it meant certain death. Humphrey recalled a moment when, in the midst of a withering firefight, an American tank got turned around and accidentally cut down its own marines. As they died by friendly fire, a fellow officer leaped up in full view of the enemy—a death sentence—and calmly used hand signals to direct the tank back toward the fight as if he were a foreman at a construction site. He lived. It was a miracle he wasn't killed instantly, one Humphrey attributed to the astonishment of the enemy.

At one point, Humphrey made a decision to save the life of a surrendering Japanese soldier—a dangerous move, considering that surrender was often used by the Japanese as a suicide ploy to blow themselves up along with their captors. He even had to face down a fellow marine who trained his own rifle on Humphrey, willing to kill him over the call. But the capture was successful and even uncovered a map—a win for army intelligence. Some fifty years later Humphrey credited that very moment with saving his humanity. With all the killing that had to be done, he jumped at the chance to save a life, even if it was the life of an enemy who might not have done the same for him. Humphrey recalled,

> On Iwo Jima it was life or death every minute of every day. There was unavoidable killing every day. When I saw that Japanese boy trying to surrender and understood that this was perhaps the only time that I didn't have to kill, I took the opportunity. *I believe that action saved my humanity.* Like most veterans of Iwo Jima who survived, I was deeply affected by the experience. But I never suffered the profound depression and shell shock (PTSD) that some of the others did. I attribute it to saving that boy's life. Protecting my enemy, if you will.[6]

Humphrey graduated Harvard Law with honors and soon found himself with a contract from the State Department's Information Service, which served as an arm of diplomacy. In 1957 the breath of the Cold War fogged international policy at a time when US-Soviet relations were on deadly footing. NATO was in Asia Minor, now Turkey, installing a region-stabilizing missile base smack in Soviet premier Nikita Khrushchev's backyard. But there was a problem—the locals. It seemed like no one wanted NATO there and protests, violence, and crime against servicefolks was rampant and rising. Humphrey's contract was to quell this unrest among the indigenous population so NATO could effectively check Soviet expansion. As Humphrey explained in his book *Values for a New Millennium*, he took a contract for two years and stayed seventeen.

Those first years were tough. The state of relations between host nationals, the American military, and its civilian contractors was unpredictable and even dangerous, with base personnel being attacked and injured. The base commander had set Humphrey straight early on in no uncertain terms: we're rich, they're poor, end of story. In his own words, the locals were dirty, smelly, stupid, thieving liars who wanted nothing more than for us to leave, or, barring that, money.

Humphrey realized his biggest obstacle wouldn't be Soviet spies but rather gaining any sense of truth—were locals really that bad? Or were these the culture-shocked thoughts of Americans used to the abundance and security of home?

The broad-brush reactions were unhelpful in dealing with the devastating poverty of the region. Tribal families lived and died in the streets and were often sick, infirm, and unclean—with no running water or sanitation to speak of, disease was rife. Revulsion too often resulted in disrespectful, even dehumanizing, attitudes—"Ugly Americanism," some would call it—one of the biggest stumbling blocks America would face to improving international relations since the end of the Great War.

Undaunted, Humphrey filled the base's Binational House with every kind of event he could think of to introduce and reintroduce host nationals to base personnel, from cocktail parties with local elites, to pot luck barbecues and cookouts, to cross-cultural exchanges such as sharing lessons on language or local customs. But they all failed miserably. At the end of his contract, Humphrey tried to dissect what went wrong—conflict was still raging.

To investigate, he did something unusual for the time and enlisted several locals to send out 2,200 surveys to get a feel for the population's concerns. It asked two questions:

1. What do you want from us Americans?
2. What can we do to improve relations?

If they really wanted money or for America to abandon their country, Humphrey secretly hoped the surveys would show it—at least it would prove he wasn't to blame. But the startling answers he received were nearly identical for both questions: *respect us as equals.*

Humphrey was thrilled—there was still hope. The systemic issues and cultural baggage on both sides could be dealt with and perhaps alleviated. Besides, Americans were the inheritors of the self-evident principles of the Declaration of Independence, that "all men are created equal." Humphrey assumed the solution was simply a standing order for the military and their civilian contractors to "show respect." End of conflict. Mission accomplished.

Confident, Humphrey called a staff meeting of the top brass to explain his findings—an unusual move for a junior officer. He methodically took everyone through the failures of his work and then to the recent surveys and suggested his standing-order fix. He argued that America's freedom was based on the equality its Founding Fathers assumed was a self-evident right. But at the end of his presentation there was no standing ovation; there was an uncomfortable, heavy silence.

It was the youngest officer, fresh from an American university, who condescendingly explained that freedom and equality were incompatible—you could have one or the other, but not both. And the Founding Fathers? They were liars—slave owners who needed a cannon fodder army to advance their own selfish interests.

The meeting devolved. The brass laid out their view: the world was teetering on the brink of nuclear war between the Soviet monster and

NATO, and the American military had an unpopular and dirty job, one that did not require getting chummy with local savages. Humphrey's superiors all but laughed him out of the room and suggested he burn his surveys. As they left, they reminded him, *animals don't deserve respect.*

Despite the drubbing, Humphrey could not let go, and he signed on for another contract. During the following months, though, his continued assertions and cross-cultural initiatives to improve relations and curb the nonstop toxic gossip and rumors about the locals fell on the deaf ears of command and were met frigidly by personnel.

Writing to his professors and mentors back home at Harvard, the Massachusetts Institute of Technology, and the Fletcher School of Diplomacy, he begged for guidance. But they could only respond with academic theories and philosophical arguments and insight—all but gobbledygook for practical use. The intellectuals had no real-world idea how to recognize and teach the concept of basic human equality as articulated in the Declaration of Independence and America's formative values.

Humphrey became despondent. His mission had failed. He had failed. He feared for the future, when the US military would be summarily kicked out of the country, the Soviets' communist machine could claim another propaganda victory, and the end of the Cold War would become still further away. To ease his mind, he got himself a hobby and started golfing—a lot. Months passed. His game improved; his attitude did not.

In the midst of his malaise, he was invited by other officers to try one of their pastimes—boar hunting. He joined military airmen in a large truck as they drove from the city into the sticks, where for pennies a day peasants would beat the brush and flush out the boars, making for a nice barbecue back at base.

The ride was like driving back in time: the city turned to countryside, which turned to villages with mud huts, mud streets, and peasants that looked as bad as they smelled. There were no sewers and no electricity, and children were surrounded by a confetti of flies.

Immediately, the negative talk started up: "Just look at these *people*."

The airmen were clearly disgusted.

"They got *nothing* to live for," one said.

"Yeah, they may as well be *dead*," another agreed.

Humphrey didn't argue. He was weary of it. Besides, it seemed true enough.

But on this day, an old army sergeant had tagged along. He was a veteran of several wars who, in dress at least, looked as rough as some of the locals. Upon hearing such talk, he drew and handed his combat knife to one of the young airmen and met his quizzical gaze with a Southern drawl: "If you think they got nothing to live for, take this knife, jump off the back of this truck, and kill one of them."

Silence. Stares.

"I've fought alongside these fellers," he continued, "and let me tell you, they kept going when plenty of Americans was yelling, 'Quit!' Maybe it's them snotty-nosed kids or women in pantaloons, but these folks value their lives just as much as we Americans do. And we have to give them that. If we don't stop talking down to them, they'll kick us out of this country."

The airmen got it. The negative talk ceased.

Humphrey's jaw dropped—this was the first time anyone had been silenced by *simple human respect*, taught practically and reasonably.

Humphrey dubbed the lesson he learned that day "The Hunting Story," and he shared it for the rest of his contract. It worked. Upon hearing it, people were struck by its plain-talking truth and simple message of equality and humility. But what Humphrey and leadership could not have predicted was that even a marginal rise in respect on behalf of the Americans was returned overwhelmingly by host nationals. Thanks in part to his work, the base stayed, the locals relaxed, and safety and morale for those stationed overseas improved.

Our Naturally Lawful Laws

Challenging the airmen, the old sergeant dares them to murder an innocent human being. Cold-blooded murder is a disvalue in modern Western society, so it's easy to imagine the short circuit it caused. The airmen's inaction exposes a deep-seated value: *respect for human life, especially innocent life.* When challenged to override this compelling inclination and adhere to what they've just claimed, they're unwilling to supersede the value of life for the sake of their opinion.

We also understand what the villagers would have done if confronted by a murderer: escape or defend themselves. This isn't even a question. The prediction of their actions is made possible by an instinctive, visceral knowledge of what we ourselves would do under the same circumstances—actions we attribute to anyone. This gut reaction reveals another underlying truth: that all human beings will instinctively protect their lives.

The old sergeant's summation as to "why they care about their lives" equates the way villagers feel about loved ones with the way we feel about ours. Even though the villagers' lifestyle is dramatically different, how could they not have the same right to exist as we do? "We have to give them that," the old sergeant said, meaning we *owe* it to them, just as they *owe* it to us—a sense of justice as a duty and service. Since all of us participate in this state of innocent human "being," in which our lives are equivalent in value, our right to exist is equal to that of anyone else. *This is as basic as basic human equality gets.*

The old sergeant would advise Humphrey that the way to deliver this simple respect to foreign cultures is to have the "guts," the courage, to put oneself at risk. This may involve getting out of one's comfort zone to try new, culturally different things or make foreign people feel more welcome. Or possibly risking one's life as law enforcement and military personnel do domestically and across the world.

By the end of the Hunting Story, we experience just what those young airmen experienced, a lesson on the inalienable right to exist that undermines any subjective belief to the contrary. The moral learned from all this is hard to deny: *our instincts recognizing the value of life as a natural truth lead us to moral truth.* It's called natural law.

You may not know of the natural law or you may know it and discount it. Some of my fellow students in grad school didn't think it was real, though it's as real as gravity. The natural law is ancient—quite the hot philosophical topic among the Greeks. It's helpful to understand it as "naturally lawful"—"natural," meaning it requires no special training to experience it, and "lawful" because it accounts for our intrinsic sense of obligations toward ourselves and others. It is often described as an explanation for why human beings obligate themselves to similar moral precepts regardless of the differences of culture—there's that universality again.

The natural law also provides for the vitality of positive law, endowing it with its sense of command and duty. In fact, when positive law becomes estranged from the touchstone of natural law, it becomes essentially unlawful. This was no more apparent than in the aftermath of World War II, when the actions of the Nazis were finally revealed to the world. During the Nuremberg trials, Nazi officers who had committed acts of unspeakable horror were to face a new concept of "crimes against humanity," since the events that occurred within concentration camps had been legal under German law. This recognition of the rights embodied within our own humanness evoked the natural law and paved the way for the 1948 United Nations Universal Declaration of Human Rights.

Natural law is also the best way to define the overused and little-understood phrase "common sense." Not to be confused with "common knowledge"—it is common knowledge that the sun will rise tomorrow—the phrase "common sense" is derived from the Latin *sensus communis*, and this from the Greek *koine aesthesis*, the "common feelings of humanity." *Cambridge Dictionary* defines it as follows: "The basic level of practical knowledge and judgment that we all need to help us live in a reasonable and safe way."[7] If this is true, there must

27

be certain nonnegotiable presuppositions "to help us live" reasonably and safely and share the "common feelings of humanity." Without this nonnegotiable aspect, which is simply another way to say "standard," how could common sense ever be *common* among us or considered wise enough to be *sensible*?

Common sense is simply this: the consistent protection, preservation, and sustainment of life in all of our actions and deeds. What is innate to our own humanness—what is naturally human—is that the value of life is the Rosetta stone that deciphers the difference between what is desirable—*subjective*—and what is necessary—*objective*—for humans. Put simply, common sense is how we have learned to refer to the natural law's "natural lawfulness" in the experience of living our lives.

For natural law to be recognized as true and universal, or, for our purposes, such that it cannot be denied, it matters not that some of us do not or will not value all life, or value everyone's lives equally. Surely we do not. Certain people's lives, including our own, matter far more to us than anyone else's, and that's normal. To be considered universal, we're not looking for everyone to value in the exact same way, but only for them to partake in *some* way. All people do not have to value all life; they only have to value *some life* to participate in *valuing* it at all, and they do—by valuing their life, or someone else's, perhaps even those of the members of their group, family, or tribe.

But since we already feel this "life value," it's reasonable to believe it could be broadened to the whole of the human community through a feeling of empathetic "common humanity" that allows us to protect ourselves and others we care about and voluntarily choose to protect the lives of strangers who cannot protect themselves.

And if we're strong enough and trained enough, we can even extend it to those who might oppose us, such as our enemies. Think about it. If, under life-and-death conditions, we could by Jedi training or genie magic protect the lives of everyone, would it be somehow offensive to our sensibilities, or our human nature? Of course not. Respect, protection, and defense of the value of life are supreme aspirations of humanity.

Without Must, Ought, and Should

The strongest argument against universal values is one made from *moral relativity*, or *relativism*, a colloquialism for the stance that there can be no truth to moral determinations and therefore there can be no objective moral values.

According to *The Stanford Encyclopedia of Philosophy*, "The term 'moral relativism' is understood in a variety of ways. Most often it is associated with an empirical thesis that there are deep and widespread moral disagreements and a metaethical thesis that the truth or justification of moral judgments is not absolute, but relative to some group of persons."[8] In other words, moral relativism argues there can be no magnetic north to the moral compass because its pull will be different throughout the world for its variety of people and cultures. It is often thought of as a "truism" due to obvious facts regarding variance in cultural values.

1. It is a fact that many cultures do not appreciate or embrace Western-style values. These values are most often described as inheritors of Athenian democratic values and progenitors of the great moral values, virtues, and standard-bearers for human rights from a Judeo-Christian ethic.
2. It is a fact that certain cultures do not embrace basic human rights as universally respectable and instead willingly treat others to the same kind of "tribalism" that they are subject to: the stoning of adulterers, the selling of children, or the dehumanizing control of women.
3. It is a fact that very often these tribal values can result in horrific indignities to the human person, and outsider tribes and cultures can be treated to violence, war, and even genocide.

29

Given these reasons and the specific instances of man's inhumanity, moral relativism is treated as a true reflection of the state of values throughout the world. But *moral relativism* is actually derived from another term, *cultural relativity*, which is intended to be understood anthropologically as a characterization of what some cultures consider to be legitimate exceptions to moral rules, but not at all as an assertion that the rules themselves do not exist.

In 1950, Clyde Kluckhohn, an American anthropologist and social scientist at Harvard University, wrote of this disparity:

> Cultural relativity means . . . that the appropriateness of any positive or negative custom must be evaluated with regard to how this habit fits with other group habits. Having several wives makes economic sense among herders, not among hunters. While breeding a healthy skepticism as to the eternity of any value prized by a particular people, anthropology does not as a matter of theory deny the existence of moral absolutes. Rather, the use of the comparative method provides a scientific means of discovering such absolutes. If all surviving societies have found it necessary to impose some of the same restrictions upon the behavior of their members, this makes a strong argument that these aspects of the moral code are indispensable.[9]

Kluckhohn makes it clear that cultural relativism as a theory is meant as a method of research and not as a theory of social or moral doctrine. He also seems to be clear that anthropology, while maintaining "healthy skepticism" about objective values, does not preclude their existence.

In his piece "The Challenge of Cultural Relativism," James Rachels outlines its impact: "Different cultures have different moral codes. What is thought right within one group may be utterly abhorrent to the members of another group, and vice versa."[10] This often leads to a mistaken notion that there can be no universal moral values. But

Rachels points out that this is not the case. In fact, there are cultural values that every culture shares—must share, in fact, or else their very existence would be threatened. Rachels states, "There is a general point here, namely, that *there are some moral rules that all societies must embrace, because those rules are necessary for society to exist.* . . . And in fact, we do find these rules in force in all cultures. Cultures may differ in what they regard as legitimate exceptions to the rules, but this disagreement exists against a background of agreement. Therefore, it is a mistake to overestimate the amount of difference between cultures. Not every moral rule can vary from society to society."[11]

Right and wrong. Good and bad. Benevolence and evil. These value claims essentially disappear when one adopts the standpoint that there are no hierarchies or absolutes concerning moral values because humanity shares no universal or objective values. This is to cede ground for judgments and value claims and adopt instead a far shakier position: opinion, where the majority or mob rules and might makes right. If you happen to be in that majority, consider yourself lucky. If you find yourself in the minority opinion, there is no ground on which to say everyone else is wrong.

Imagine fifty people enter a room and declare a thing as moral. And then fifty-one other people enter the same room and declare that not only is that thing immoral, the first fifty people should be killed. If majority rules, and opinion itself is the fulcrum of moral weight, on what ground can the first fifty people claim the fifty-one are wrong? Human agreement is a flawed way of determining moral validity because human reasoning is not always "reasonable." Gordon Graham concurs in his *Theories of Ethics*:

The policy of genocide was not made wrong by the post war agreement of the Allies. Its wrongness transcends all such agreements. This is why the word "bad" seems so inadequate and why the word "evil" seems indispensable. It is also what the language of "crimes against humanity" is intended to capture. And yet this too seems to accomplish nothing. If one set of human beings (e.g., the Nazis or the Allies) cannot make these things right or wrong, neither can humanity as a whole. Should the whole of humanity accept something unjust as just (as it once accepted the institution of slavery), this would not *make* it just; it would only show how degraded human beings had become.[12]

When we adopt the standpoint of relativism, we then reject the standard of basic value claims. This is because metaphysical notions of oughtness can only exist when there is recognition that the value of life provides the justification for any and all claims of how we "must, ought, or should." Without that justification, these words are mere suggestions and hold no command. Instead, we embrace a state of the world in which there can be no true right and wrong. Just like the misguided notion "Beauty is in the eye of the beholder," "goodness" and "evil" are merely in the eye of theirs.

On its face the argument from moral relativity is inherently untrue (and contradictory) for it stipulates a generalization it cannot possibly prove. It says, in effect, that due to the presence of specific individual examples, a true generalization can be made. In essence, it makes the following argument:

Because values vary from culture to culture, it must be true that there are no objective moral values that are universal for all people.

Here's an analogical argument concerning food:

Because cooking varies from culture to culture, it must be true that there can be no single dish that is nourishing for all people.

Perhaps there is no single dish that will entice the tastes of all people, but that's not at issue. It's the contention that there can be no way to nourish all people with a single dish. Of course, we know this to be false—all food, provided it is food, nourishes the human body. Unless folks were born on the planet Mars and have acid for blood, there is no doubt food provides nourishment for them.

Because the moral values aim at the protection and respect of cultures and societies and not against them, there are always going to be limitations on the variances of moral codes from culture to culture. Moral relativism as cultural relativity should in no way promote the notion that universal moral codes fundamental to the protection, sustainment, and respect of the value of life themselves cannot or do not exist.

The Polite Absurdity

Although moral relativism is often portrayed as an intrinsically humble approach to foreign cultures and creeds it actually taps into and cultivates a palpable sense of nihilism. Claiming one can have no true moral knowledge is to claim there is no such thing as moral truth—a nihilistic ideal.

Nihilism asserts itself as a purely destructive force; it denounces belief in all values and relinquishes participation in social, political, and religious institutions, claiming they are challenges to personal freedom. The concept is also associated with "ethical" and "existential" conceptions that posit there can be no truth in moral or ethical decision making and behavior, as well as no value to be found in life whatsoever. "Nothing matters" is the essential mantra of nihilism. And once this belief takes firm hold, and no value can be assigned to life itself, its logical conclusion is not far behind: "No one matters"—the clarion call of dehumanization.

When comedians Mel Brooks and Carl Reiner performed the "2000 Year Old Man" sketch, they touched on a sensitive truth:

BROOKS: We had a national anthem.
REINER: What was the anthem?

BROOKS: Well, you see, it was very fragmented. It wasn't a nation. It was caves. Each cave had a national anthem.

REINER: Do you remember the national anthem of your cave?

BROOKS: I certainly do. I'll never forget. You never forget a national anthem in a minute. [Singing] *Let 'em all go to hell! Except cave 76!*

Dehumanization is the devastating removal of respect and human dignity throughout history from those deemed "subhuman" in order to transform them into merchandise, property, or mere targets for destruction.

The concept is toxic for two central reasons:

1. It can seem like an impenetrable shield.
2. It can be a seductive, easily employed weapon.

By treating everyone outside one's group as a potential enemy, dehumanization can provide the feeling one is "protecting" one's group and oneself, enforcing security rather than destabilizing it by disrespecting others. A shared obligation of both civilian leadership and civil and military protectors is to examine the training, teaching, and shaping of ethics to best emulate and embody common values. It should establish a defense against the seduction of dehumanization's shield that can itself feel like inoculation against the various kinds of culture and poverty shock experienced in worldwide theaters, as well as on the domestic front in dealing with the least of us.

But as a weapon to use against one's enemies, dehumanization is much worse. By focusing on brutal behavior—perhaps perpetrated by only a few—in conflict and atrocities, playing up stereotypes, or emphasizing what may be considered strange cultural affectations, enemies can be made to appear subhuman, which places them on par with the animal world, and therefore makes them easier to kill. Propaganda efforts among the Hutu administration were busy dehumanizing their Tutsi neighbors as early as 1990. Ramping up tribal fervor before genocide in 1994, Tutsis were referred to as "cockroaches," and calls for violence became comprehensive. Jonathan Glover points this out in his book *Humanity*:

> Tribal hostility is the obvious powerful emotion and Rwanda looks like a classic case of traditional tribal hatred erupting into massacre. The emotion is correctly identified, but it is too simple to think of it as either "traditional" or as just "erupting." . . . The tribes were not sharply divided. They spoke the same language, had a shared culture and there were many marriages between [them]. . . . The genocide was not a spontaneous eruption of tribal hatred, it was planned by people wanting to keep power. There was a long government-led hate campaign against the Tutsis. In 1990 the journal *Kangura* published "The Hutu Ten Commandments," one of which said that any Hutu who married, employed or even befriended a Tutsi woman was a traitor. . . . A Hutu [radio] station owned by relatives of the President, poured out propaganda against the Tutsis. . . . After [the president's death was blamed on the Tutsis] the radio station urged killing Tutsis. . . . Children were included. The human responses were overwhelmed in the killers by tribal hatred, but this emotion was itself a product of conscious political manipulation.[13]

Dehumanization can also be self-imposed. When compassion and empathy cause regular folks to risk their own and others' safety so as not to hurt the feelings of others, we have reached what I call the "polite absurdity." It's not just the drive to force solutions to problems out of everyone's practical control—anyone can slap a fresh coat of paint on a ramshackle home to make it look more accommodating. But placing oneself in needless jeopardy—tacit dehumanization—for the sake of someone else's feelings is more like painting that shack as it burns itself to the ground.

Case in point: the polite absurdity was on stunning display in November 2014 with the story of Oliver Friedfeld, the young Georgetown University student who wrote the piece "I Was Mugged, and

I Understand Why" after he was actually mugged on campus at gunpoint.

This young man not only didn't blame his attackers but also ascribed to them nonviolent motives, which, of course, is a contradiction, because when your life is threatened—leveraged toward your compliance against the menace of harm—the motive is necessarily violent.

Friedfeld advised the rest of us to "get comfortable" with the occasional mugging and break-in. He declared in his piece, "Who am I to stand from my perch of privilege, surrounded by million-dollar homes and paying for a $60,000 education, to condemn these young men as 'thugs'? It's precisely this kind of 'otherization' that fuels the problem."[14]

Who is he? An equal human being, that's who. Even from his so-called perch of privilege. Friedfeld's life is not worth less just because he has more. I suspect he does not see the irony of his statement, which is that his muggers actually "otherized" him—read, *dehumanized*—as they were threatening to murder him had he not obeyed their wishes. That's more of an offense than merely acknowledging "thuggery" makes one a "thug" regardless of race.

I don't blame Friedfeld for not condemning his assailants; he's afflicted with moral relativism, which trains people to blind themselves to truth in moral conclusions. Its symptom is ethical befuddlement and, worse, apathy—the conscious choice to stop caring about protecting oneself and others.

If Friedfeld truly believes his life is not worthy of the basic level of respect that demands it not be placed under threat of murder, then he's all the synonyms listed in Microsoft Word's thesaurus for *appallingly*—such as *frighteningly, horrifyingly, terrifyingly*, and *shockingly*—confused. We must always temper our compassion and empathy with the responsibility to protect ourselves and others, even when we are trying to protect our enemy. And we should not take advantage of ourselves by taking our own safety for granted in the hope we won't offend the feelings of others. It's always a poor idea to obscure truth, especially to defend some imagined moral high ground, because the high ground is only useful if it's *actually* the high ground and not merely ground we declare to be high.

Though virtue aims at the good, it doesn't always get there, thus its challenge. And sometimes, with all the best intentions, it can go wildly off course. Take Friedfeld's empathy. Now, empathy is a necessary component to understand not just the needs and wants of others but also ourselves. Our empathetic drives steer us to be both reflective of how we ourselves wish to be treated in similar contexts, and reflexive about our actions and their impact on others. Empathy is necessary to authenticate the experience of our Golden Ruled common humanity, be it with people we care about or strangers in a strange land.

Because empathy arises from our inherent natural law, it occurs without a lot of conscious work on our part. But that doesn't mean there are not plenty of folks clocking overtime for it, resulting in *too much empathy*. If we can express too little, we can certainly express too much, and too much, like too little, doesn't look or sound or act much like empathy at all. We can force ourselves to empathize with other people too much, in spite of our best intentions.

Aristotle had a genius way of looking at this disparity. He figured that all virtue was under a "doctrine of the mean," a principle that took the application of virtue as roughly the balance between its excess and deficiency, both vices to Aristotle. Courage was the mean between its "too much," foolhardiness, and its "too little," cowardice. Many of the virtues we find appealing backfire when they exceed this mandate. "Too much of anything is bad," Mark Twain said, "but too much good whiskey is barely enough." Insofar as good whiskey is one of my favorite virtues—"water of life" and all—too much empathy is not "barely enough"—it is realistically no longer empathy.

It's easy to see deficiency here, or at least easier than it is to see excess. Too little empathy is apathetic and egoistic and, quite frankly, dishonest, in terms of the rights and duties we have toward the lives of others. We might call it "cold-hearted"—a selfish take that places us above others and says, "What is good for me is not good for them." Now, this may or may not have adverse effects. Inaction under given circumstances is still an action, but it may not result in poor consequences for oneself or others.

However, the excess is worse, primarily because it does adversely affect our self-image. Too much empathy drives us toward a selflessness that is ignorant of the rights and duties we have toward ourselves. It says, in effect, "What is good for them is also good for me." Now, this is great if you're talking shared human rights, but it's not so great if you're empowering others to strip yours rights away. Too much selfless empathy makes us naïve by dulling our self-respect, numbing us to the expectations of moral and ethical behavior of others. Worse, it can lead to fanaticism, where one willingly equates their objective value of life with the subjective whims of others. This is to become a moral cultist, eager to sacrifice the self to satisfy the banal demands of those who would make such demands. It flips truth on its head and is a terrifying outcome toward the drive to do good.

Our senses speak to us as a voice of collected experiences, context, environment, and variables, informing us that we ought not disrespect ourselves by dropping any pretense of self-worth before or after such harrowing experiences, like being mugged. Nobody has the right to take advantage of us or anyone we love or care about—our lives are just as valuable to us as any offender's is to him or her.

We ought not think of ourselves unethically, due to post-traumatic stress, by believing there is no blame to assign for a crime committed against us and, by that logic, no crime committed. It is a lie to think this, for it shakes and weakens the very values folks like Friedfeld no doubt place great faith in, such as fairness and equality—what's fair or equal about having violence forced on you and against your better interests?

What more can justify and authenticate such lofty values if the value we hold for our lives is so meaningless that we will not speak against being arbitrarily harmed for the money in our pockets by those twisted enough to threaten violence for it? Folks like Friedfeld are so morally adrift they're unwilling to stand up for even the dignity of their own lives by condemning violent actions upon them as immoral and unethical. It is exactly this kind of appeasement that ensures those crimes will proliferate and reinforces to both the perpetrators and their victims that the use of such unjust force is perfectly justifiable because it's all for the sake of "justice."

To know a crime was committed, to assign blame, to name the thug as anyone who engages in thuggery, is to pay homage to and keep sacred the concept of self-respect and not allow arbitrary, relative concerns—such as desire, greed, poverty's desperation, or our compassion and empathy, for that matter—to supersede in importance this universal connection of our common humanity.

To believe otherwise is to lie to oneself and disorient from truth.

It is to be mugged and not understand why.

Calibrating the Moral Compass

The value of life involves two distinct aspects: the physical—life itself or the actual human "being" of aliveness—and the metaphysical in orbit around it that is everything we consider worthwhile in life—our loves, ambitions, and desires, including our sense of oughtness referenced within morals, ethics, justice, and rights.

This physical and metaphysical are so closely aligned, similar to how the moon orbits Earth, that it's difficult to separate them. Who sees life as only about being alive? No one. We *live* in our lives, living for, and with hopeful anticipation of, its many goods. What's clear is that metaphysical concerns are *only* important because life itself is so vital.

Yes, the moon imparts an influence on Earth; however, without Earth to orbit, why would that influence matter? It couldn't. So it wouldn't. Without life to impact, the metaphysical aspects that humanity considers worthwhile do not matter. There is no love or forgiveness; no passion, joy, or happiness; no kindness, compassion, or grace; no humility, gratitude, or even wonder regarding these processes without humanity's corporeal body, the actual vessel for these feelings, emotions, thoughts, and concerns to take place in and thrive, so we can emote them to others. They only matter if we're around to live them.

This small logic may seem rather boring or inchoate. But, in terms of moral epistemic veracity, it stands out like Carmen Miranda singing "Chica Chica Boom Chic" under fireworks because it opens the door to moral truth and just how we can know it.

Moral truth is simply this: *protect respect for the value of life and don't disrespect it for subjective concerns.* It's not revolutionary, except when you put it in context against what many believe are the highest values of society. Whichever you might choose as the pinnacle of ethical endeavor, its particular formulation can only.be truthfully moral if it does not disrespect or encroach on life for relative concerns. This means, in essence, that in order to qualify as moral, metaphysical values must respect the value of life. If they do not, or when they do not, then you most assuredly have something immoral.

Now some will claim this is too problematic, for if protection of life is to be the ultimate moral standard, we're looking at something terribly impractical, as we'll have to outlaw driving and processed foods and *Star Wars* Christmas specials since they endanger life far too much, as well as any conception of "just war" or self-defense, since there will always be the chance of an enemy's life being taken.

But this is misguided. Folks can cause all kinds of havoc when they align their ethical destination with the literal justifier of the moral compass, which would be similar to traveling to a magnetic pole—north or south, it's awfully cold.

In terms of ethics, this disordering leads good folks to misinterpret the waypoints of their journey as signs they are heading in the right direction, when they are actually being led to chaos. Pacifism makes the claim that the value of human life is its highest ideal, so much so that it affirms that life must never be violently harmed under any circumstance. And yet, to be unwilling to protect innocent human life from violent harm is actually about maintaining dedication to one's personal autonomy. This has the effect of replacing pacifism's supposedly highest ideal with an idle concern—a fatal contradiction.

The worst part is that pacifism, contrary to its marketing, is not an empowerment of the loftiest aspirations of the human condition; it is the surrender of them to any fight whatever, even before that fight decides to take a swing. And don't mistake pacifism here for nonviolent resistance—there is nothing passive whatever about risking oneself to stand for basic human rights in the face of threats of danger. The pacifist I speak of stays home in forfeit.

To correctly use a compass, at least three rules must be followed:

1. We must identify and recognize a true magnetic pole—in the Northern Hemisphere, this is magnetic north.
2. We must then identify and orient to our destination by direction and thereby set a bearing. This ensures accuracy so we can get to where we want to go.
3. In traveling toward our destination, we must negotiate the actual terrain before us as best we can, and in accordance with the directional bearing we've set through alignment to the magnetic pole, so as not to deviate from our course.

Anytime we use a compass, even the moral compass, the magnetic pole is never our destination—unless you're a scientist or a bearded eighteenth-century explorer trying to win an ill-conceived bet. The pole's steadfast value creates a standard to maintain a bearing to calibrate by as we navigate toward our actual destination. That's the function of its standard. Without it, navigation is unreliable.

It should be noted that morality evolves and does in fact change—even the ghastly institution of slavery was at one time predominately considered moral and just around the world. Does this evolving morality mean that any of the moral notions we might have today are by default the best because they are the latest, most fashionable, shiniest models?

No, not in the least.

Imagine a time in the future when the world's mad scientists, aided by melon-headed aliens from a crazy-advanced alternative dimension, create a plant-based food just as tasty as meat, in a million years or so, and using magic. This meatless future could drive a moral trend that pronounces meat eating and meat products to be immoral and then retro-assess that at any time people ate meat, raised animals for food, hunted, and used leather products—much like today—they were immoral for doing so.

It's important to remember that morals often correspond to their generation. Due to the molten rock swirling beneath Earth's crust, the magnetic North and South Poles shift around and can actually switch polarity. As such, they are not the geographic poles found on maps—they move around too much. The topography of the land also changes, as do compass bearings and directions. All of this is a natural result of the impact of time, gravity, and the features of age. But among all of these fluctuating aspects, the poles remain magnetized. In other words, claims of morality may change, as well as how we might arrive at moral conclusions, but the reason we have morals at all—why morals matter in the first place—does not change: *the value of life is immutably valuable.*

For true justice, we must start with recognition of this natural truth, accept it, and assess all other relative concerns against it. There is no subjective value that justifies innocent human life and validates it as relevant and meaningful. If there were, then it would be perfectly justifiable to threaten, harm, and murder an innocent human being for the "sake" of that stated value. If freedom, liberty, or democracy were more important than the objective value of life, then mowing down innocents with a truck would be a perfectly justifiable way to achieve it. Swap out for any other concern and the answer is just as bleak.

When we do not adhere to this reality and instead invent perceptions that do not exist, we can wind up accepting notions that do in fact "justify" life. And in that confusion we can accept ideologies, organizations, governments, or opinions, as trendy as any fashion cat-walk, that willfully challenges and seeks to dictate an alternative to our intrinsic dignity.

Honor

Martial training takes certain things for granted. If it did not, it could not exist. For instance: life has value and meaning. And that value and meaning are unequivocal. In other words, it is the normative source of all the concerns we might have in navigating the world, including decisions regarding morals and ethics. And when that compass needle deviates from that central concern, everything gets confusing.

All people who train and endeavor to train must understand, at least on some basic level, that life is worth protecting. If they did not think this, why train physically to protect it? If you believe that only some life is worth protecting because some life is deemed dignified, then martial training cannot be fulfilled. How could we possibly apply that notion to strangers? We can't know whether a person is a saint or a son of a bitch.

The concern here is that there is no shortage of subjectivity. And when these relative concerns supersede universal ones, we're left with contradictions that stoke conflict. Take freedom and equality—these mutually exclusive concepts protect each other, as our founders discovered. We are all born equal human beings and should be treated respect-fully. As a universal value, that means no one has the right to take advantage of, harm, or kill us for relative beliefs. Freedom is the lib-erty to pursue whichever relative beliefs we find valuable, *provided* they do not violate our universal equality—respect for the value of life. These concepts complement each other and share a nice balance between them, as their purpose is contingent on such balance.

But if we redefine equality as pertaining not to life but to "outcome," a subjective economic concern in which everyone must receive the same results, no matter what they want, who they want it from, or what values they might conflict with, we wind up out of balance and lose our freedom. Redefine equality not as a universal but a relative value and it is no longer compatible with freedom. Equality and freedom then become just arbitrary concerns competing with other arbitrary concerns. It inevitably causes conflict by violating people's liberty if they cannot side with their own values when they conflict with other people's values. Equality of outcome means uniform results—*your values be damned*.

Without equality being defined universally, we cannot enjoy our relative freedom. And when an individual, group, or a state-sponsored entity, compels us through force to do something we would never voluntarily do, such as engage with others and participate in ways that are antithetical to our values—values that are not in violation of equality of life—then we are being taken advantage of. And if we are being taken advantage of, we are certainly not being treated as equal human beings.

True justice results in equality as a service to your fellow man and gives us a just way to live. By obeying our inherent natural law to do what we say we will do and refrain from encroaching on others, we fulfill the duties to ourselves as well as others. Basic to the martial way is the understanding that the value of life is our sense of self-worth and self-risk. No matter where you stand politically, or what your beliefs are, if you embrace the protector ethic, then you embrace the idea that life is worth protecting and defending. So no matter how far you believe people with the opposite set of beliefs or politics or values stand from you, you are not as far away from them, or they from you, as you might think.

The martial way is simply a physical extension of our natural law. Training gives us a sturdier sense of that obligation, reenforcing the fact that it is worth protecting, and because it is worth protecting, it is worth defending physically if necessary.

All the questions we might have about whether people are equal to each other, whether we should treat each other fairly, and how we should understand each other come down to the justification of our argument—does it respect the value of life?

If so, then we can value the right morals, articulate the right reasons, protect the right rights, act on the right ethics, and aspire to the right virtues, all because we're dialed in to true justice. Everything hinges on it.

This is where honor comes from.

Constancy in acting on this makes one honorable.

NOTES

1. Immanuel Kant, *Groundwork for the Metaphysics of Morals*, trans. Mary Gregor (New York: Cambridge University Press, 2007), 30.
2. Mark Twain, *Plymouth Rock and the Pilgrims and Other Salutary Platform Opinions*, ed. Charles Neider (New York: Harper and Row, 1984), 309.
3. C. W. Nevius, "Veterans Share Views on Iraq War," *SFGATE*, December 13, 2005.
4. Karl M. Petruso, "Early Weights and Weighing in Egypt and the Indus Valley," *M Bulletin* (Museum of Fine Arts, Boston) 79 (1981): 45.
5. M. I. Finley, *The World of Odysseus*, introduction by Simon Hornblower (London: Folio Society, 2002), 76.
6. Quoted in Jack Hoban, *The Ethical Warrior* (Spring Lake, NJ: RGI Media and Publications, 2012), 123 (emphasis in the original).
7. *Cambridge Dictionary*, 4th ed., s.v. "common sense," accessed September 6, 2017, http://dictionary.cambridge.org/us/dictionary/english/common-sense.
8. Chris Gowans, "Moral Relativism," in *The Stanford Encyclopedia of Philosophy*, winter 2016 ed., ed. Edward N. Zalta, https://plato.stanford.edu/archives/win2016/entries/moral-relativism/.
9. Clyde Kluckhohn, *Mirror for Man: The Relation of Anthropology to Modern Life* (London: George G. Harrap, 1950).
10. James Rachels, "The Challenge of Cultural Relativism," in *The Elements of Moral Philosophy*, 6th ed., ed. Stuart Rachels (Boston: McGraw Hill, 2010), 14.
11. Ibid., 23 (emphasis in the original).
12. Gordon Graham, *Theories of Ethics* (New York: Routledge, 2011), 136.

13. Jonathan Glover, *Humanity: A Moral History of the Twentieth Century* (New Haven, CT: Yale University Press, 1999), 121.
14. Oliver Friedfeld, "I Was Mugged, and I Understand Why," *Hoya*, November 18, 2014, http://www.thehoya.com/i-was-mugged-and-i-understand-why/.

2

To Reason: Temperance as Integrity

Stepping Forward

On November 21, 2009, Gerardo Sanchez, an exterminator living in New York, stepped aboard a D train and started acting crazy. He confronted a drifter over a seat when plenty were available, pulled a knife, and stabbed the man repeatedly in his neck and face, slashing his carotid artery. He did this in front of dozens of terrified passengers. The victim died at the scene and, eerily, still in his seat, with his eyes open. But what happened next is the creepy part.

After passengers pulled the emergency brake and reported the crime to the conductor, the train car was locked down—sealed—from the outside. And now this group of passengers, innocents all, was confined with a bloodied killer, the knife still in his hand.

Where would you have placed yourself in that moment? Stuffed into the huddled mass of people seeking shelter from a killer? Or in front, positioned between the killer and others? Luckily, Sanchez pried open one of the train car doors just enough to drop the knife onto the tracks. No one else was hurt.

Self-risk must be a bold, conscious choice. Unless it is, we cannot think of ourselves as protectors. In training, the person we always learn to defend first is ourselves, for if we cannot or will not protect ourselves, we're unlikely to protect anyone else. In college, a fellow philosophy student was a high-ranking exponent of a Korean martial art, and he was quite good at it. In fact, I remember watching him in astonishment as he sprinted, momentarily, across a padded wall—a feat of balance and speed. But he also enjoyed explaining to me that as a pacifist, he was not willing to use his martial training to defend even himself. At the time, I remember thinking, "Then what's the point?" Of course, what I hear today in his statement is that he's dedicated himself to mastering CPR, but under no conditions would he use its knowledge or skills to protect human life.

Knowing martial arts is not enough. At advanced levels, training is not about anticipating when an opponent will strike, but *enduring the moment we have allowed them to do so.* Communicating an opening, a vulnerability, one they can scarcely ignore, fulfills their intent and empowers with the thrill of easy advantage. This self-sacrifice is one of the most difficult martial efforts because it places us at greater risk to fulfill our ethic and do the right thing. This, in turn, challenges us to be more physically able, and it all starts with the choice to risk.

Temperance is the virtue known as restraint. "Wherefore temperance takes the need of this life, as the rule of the pleasurable objects of which it makes use, and uses them only for as much as the need of this life requires," says Thomas Aquinas in his *Summa Theologica.* Martial artists know it as self-control. Whether in thought, word, or deed, it's the general mind-set for behavior.

In short, we care. We care about the consequences of our actions, which is why self-control is really about our own sense of self-respect and self-worth. How well we respect ourselves contributes mightily to how well we control ourselves. And how well we control ourselves, our integrity, determines whether we can reason to risk and sacrifice for others.

Self-Risk Is Self-Worth

The first thing Brian Nichols did to escape from the Fulton County courthouse was beat a five-foot, fifty-one-year-old sheriff's deputy into a coma. She would later become an invalid, unable to testify against him. Stealing her gun, he stormed the courtroom where he was on trial for rape and executed his judge, along with a court reporter who just happened to be there. He searched for his two prosecutors and the woman he raped, but, unable to find them, he fled, killing a pursuing police officer. On the streets, Nichols carjacked several people, smashing some with the butt of his gun, and tried to kidnap others. He would commit at least fifty-four crimes.

On March 11, 2005, roadblocks shut down Atlanta, Georgia, as squad cars, helicopters, a hundred state troopers, and the FBI joined the manhunt. That night, Nichols ambushed a federal agent in his own home as he tiled his bathroom floor and stole his truck. It would be the last life he would take.

Nichols then took hostage Ashley Smith, a drug-addicted single mother trying to turn herself around. Giving Nichols her last bit of crystal meth, Smith, a Christian, spoke of her daughter, whom she was scheduled to see that day. She read passages from the Bible to him, along with Pastor Rick Warren's *Purpose Driven Life*, and even made him pancakes when he was hungry. It worked. Nichols repented and allowed Smith to leave, after which she called police. A SWAT team arrested Nichols shortly after he emerged from Smith's apartment waving a white flag. He's now serving multiple life sentences.

Nichols was clearly bloodthirsty, but Smith was smart, giving up the drugs he wanted and humanizing herself, thus granting an opportunity to escape. Perhaps it was fate or luck, but Smith did something many might not have done: she risked to protect her aggressor, because protecting him meant protecting herself. She reasoned first by the ethical, and that gave her a tactical advantage.

When we reason, we aren't comparing and deciding things, as we do when judging. Reason identifies the choices that we will later judge to act on. If you've ever said, "Be reasonable," or you've been told you're "not being reasonable," this is referencing overlooked choices believed to be sensible considerations.

The best-known reasoning model is MAUA, the Multi-attribute Utility and Decision Analysis. It generates wide options, identifies criteria to evaluate, assigns weight, and tabulates scores for maximum and minimum outcomes. Yet according to studies dating back to the 1960s, most people are actually poor reasoners, failing even simple logical tasks—as if we needed fifty years of studies to confirm this.

Personal biases sway our thinking. Experiences, environment, the way in which we inform ourselves, and the extent to which we are informed create *intuitions*, which generally enforce the biases we had to begin with. Evolutionary psychologists mark a distinction between intuitive inferences and cognitive reasoning simply because how people reason is not always connected to reality but is often the result of its perception. In effect, we want to confirm our biases. Dr. Raymond S. Nickerson called it the "seeking or interpreting of evidence in ways that are partial to existing beliefs, expectations, or a hypothesis in hand."[1]

But MAUA fails in real-world, complex settings, in which time, stress, and rapidly changing conditions are inescapable, such as in conflict, fighting, and life-and-death stuff. Turns out, when experienced protectors act, they don't make a list of pros and cons first.

Field researchers chronicled firefighting, rescue, and even battle planning, in which participants were extensively trained, and discovered that once on scene, gone were the endless maximizations. Instead, participants engaged in *satisficing*, or accepting available options. Called RPD, recognition-primed decisions, it accepts the burden of changing situations, real-time reactions, pressures, task conditions, and, most importantly, the consequences of mistakes, and, I would add, of successes—there's no assurance that even when everything is done right, lives will not be lost. The most important feature of RPD: recognizing and classifying situations based on prior training. And therein lies the key: *context*.

If martial training is about anything, it's not simply about practicing a range of techniques as options; rather, it's about habit forming a method to shape those options for given moments. This means even one technique could be utilized in a variety of ways under a variety of conditions. To understand this, we have to recognize the undeniable: *ethics beget tactics*. The most ethical choice we can satisfice, or accept under real-world conditions, will always inform us of the surest tactical action we can take.

Reason to Risk

Tactics do not beget ethics. We could take any number of tactical actions—none of them may be ethical. But if we identify the most ethical choice we can satisfice in a given situation, we will automatically be directed to the most tactical action we can perform.

Remember, we're out to identify two aspects: (1) what we *ought* to do; and, based on this, (2) what we are *capable of doing*.

Keep in mind, this choice may not actually be the "most ethical" or "most tactical" because we may simply not be capable of these actions in a particular moment for a variety of reasons. Yes, I would prefer to save all the puppies that are drowning, but in reality I can save only a couple without drowning myself. Context will inform us. How do we know? Simple: remove from the equation the ethical choice to risk oneself and tactical options drastically diminish. But place ourselves in the mix and they improve.

To better think like a protector, we should know what it means to not think like one. This ethical problem is an excerpt by Elizabeth

Ashford and Tim Mulgan from *The Stanford Encyclopedia of Philosophy*:

The Rocks

Six innocent swimmers have become trapped on two rocks by the incoming tide. Five of the swimmers are on one rock, while the last swimmer is on the second rock. Each swimmer will drown unless they are rescued. You are the sole life-guard on duty. You have time to get to one rock in your patrol boat and save everyone on it. Because of the distance between the rocks, and the speed of the tide, you cannot get to both rocks in time.

What should you do?[2]

Now, their proposed solution is to toss a coin. Seriously. Look it up. That way each person has a fair possibility of being rescued because they're given a fifty-fifty chance at rescue. I love this—lives literally hang in the balance, and they decide that randomness will dictate their actions. Two-Face, the villain from Batman comics, flips a coin to decide who lives and who dies—*a comic book character*. This is just the kind of incompatible-with-real-life answer that outlines the problem for modern philosophy. When folks look to it for nourishment, they're often fed exotic appetizers rather than a hearty meal—forget Thanksgiving dinner, it's *balut* with roasted beetles for you.

There are lots of ways to problem solve in ethics: person-to-person virtue ethics, in which we ask if we are the kind of person who does the act in question, or deontological methods, which are a kind of principlism that relies on rules to define behavior, like a casuistry for case-to-case comparisons. Too often, though, I find academic ethics relying on moral gerrymandering meant to indoctrinate students with a kind of consequentialist—read, utilitarian—heuristic of *aggregation* to save the five and sacrifice the one.

Utilitarianism is the pleasure-pain philosophy of John Stuart Mill that advocates the greatest good for the greatest number. At first, this may sound like a good, reasonable thing—more is always more than less. We like to aggregate all kinds of stuff, such as money, time, and energy, so why not do it with human well-being? Pop culture has also ingrained the notion. The most memorable scene from *Star Trek* is when Captain Kirk loses his second and otherwise BFF, Spock. In *The Wrath of Khan*, after sacrificing himself to save the ship and crew, Spock dies inside a radiation chamber and bonds with his old friend through a protective door, rasping, "The needs of the many . . ." "Outweigh the needs of the few," breaks Kirk. "Or the one," Spock whispers.

But it's worth mentioning that this pithy saying could be used to justify horrific "needs of the many" such as slavery and genocide, since, without qualification, definitions are always open to interpretation. Ari Armstrong of *The Objective Standard* points out, "Which 'many'? Which 'few'? 'Outweigh' on whose scale? For what purpose? To whose benefit? Why is his or their benefit the proper benefit?" And here's me nerding out loud: Did Spock *really* put the "needs of the many" above his few? His sacrifice was an eminently reasonable decision, especially considering that he alone had the resilience and training to withstand death itself—he's half-alien, didn't exactly die, and ensured he wouldn't by transferring his consciousness into Dr. McCoy. In fact, see the follow-up, *Star Trek: The Search for Spock*, in which, funny enough, the needs of the one—Spock—outweigh the needs of the many, the USS *Enterprise* crew, who break rank and struggle to rescue him.

Though the coin toss solution to our rocks question avoids aggregation, it offers the equally bleak solution of indiscriminate—indifferent to differences—chance. But when we avoid identifying the difference between what we aspire to do and what we can do it dramatically affects our actions by *reducing* our options. "More options" sounds like "more freedom" to me than less, and freedom in action is a good, especially if you're in the business of saving lives. The professors have placed the tactical—use of the coin—over the ethical *context* of the situation itself. And placing tactics before ethics does not get you ethical answers to ethical questions. It gets you awful tactics.

What the professors are overlooking in their problem are two important aspects of context: one of obligation and one of value. The original iteration states, "You are the sole life-guard." This represents cultivated physical ability and an *obligation* toward others to protect them. It is indicative of the fact that one is trained as an expert rescue swimmer to protect others from drowning. Also, if each of these people has an equal claim to be rescued, and they do, then it's because their lives are of equal worth and value, and that is exactly what is implied: each rock-clinging soul keeps from dying by clinging to the rocks. When these two points are not overlooked, there are now more choices to make our action more ethical.[3]

I say drive the boat toward the rock with the five. When they can reach it, dive into the turbulent water to attempt a rescue of the sixth swimmer. The five can share responsibility to save themselves and have an opportunity to work together to do so—unlike the solo swimmer—using the boat to keep each other afloat and save one another. At that time, they could even drive the boat to pick up the sixth swimmer and you. Even if the sixth swimmer slips into the water and drowns, the chances of recovering and reviving that single person are better than all six at the same time.

The only common sense these professors inadvertently discover with their explanation is that there is value to life and we ought to protect it—the fact that they advocate flipping a coin *at all* proves they feel obligated to do something over nothing. A coin toss is a fine way to see which team kicks off because it epitomizes the Latin *ceteris paribus*, which we know well as "all things being equal," meaning there are no factors or circumstances that might cause one to believe things are not equal. But our responsibility to ourselves and others will always entail factors and circumstances—*context*—that mightily contradict "all things being equal" for the simple reason that they never, ever, ever are.

Context matters because context *always* matters. Can you name a decision made without reflective input from its conditions? Why are you there? Who are you and what's your role in all this? Who are these people on the rocks? Do you know any? How is it happening and how quickly is it unfolding? These aspects aren't minor; they impact the final question, namely, "What should I do?"—*the* question of ethical questions. The coin flip for life or death is not an ethical choice and would be laughable if it were not so insulting. Just the act of advocating it is another indicator of the tacit appeal to apathy.

When we refuse to discipline our behavior by way of virtue, we make it easier to tap the vein of apathy that lies just below the surface of our psyche. We stop caring. And when we stop caring, we can conclude that a coin flip to determine who goes home and who doesn't is just dandy, and we can even compose lengthy diatribes to defend it. Apathy is unrestrained—it has no reason for self-control because it doesn't care about consequences and how they might affect others. Apathy condemns. It revokes any duty to identify the moral.

Self-control through martial training is how to reason like a protector precisely because it comes from disciplined self-risking. The professors fail to acknowledge that even though their coin indicates who will survive, it also condemns who will not. It is as much a death dealer as it is a life giver. Sorry, but I prefer my moral actions to be actually moral, where life protecting is the name of the game and not just a happy accident.

Self-risk in our reasoning is all geared toward a singular ideal: making better judgments and decisions, an aspect of prudence. Protectors must recognize and intuit the kind of ethical insight necessary to identify better tactical choices. Training should not break down into specific "what-to-dos"—techniques—but rather habituate moral choices so we can shape those techniques under given circumstances. The ethical context will always speak to its actionable options.

When boots touch down and it's the individual who must reason, judge, and act, the utilitarian maximization of "the good" often fails when applied to *you-tilitarian* values, such as when that one straggler clinging to yonder rock is the very person most important to you—there's that *context* again. And then we might as well backhand that stupid coin into the Trevi for luck.

✳ The Moral as Martial: Discipline

When I was a boy, a kid I'd never seen before rode up next to me and said, "Nice bike!"

It was. A Mongoose—yellow frame, black trim, squishy grips I can still feel to this day.

I looked him over. He was wearing a white tank-top undershirt and riding a scratched-up bike with a banana seat and chopper handlebars. Not exactly the height of cool.

I instinctively knew he wasn't from around here. Maybe he was from Berwyn, a decidedly tougher area than the "Village in the Forest," Riverside, Illinois. But it was the compliment that pinged my radar. Nine-year-old strangers in my day didn't compliment; we scowled—a defense mechanism to protect our fragile sense of cool, whatever that was.

"Thanks," I finally said, but clearly meaning, "What sit ta you?"

What it was to him was kung fu-ing my back tire, sending me flying off my sweet ride to eat curb. I scraped up my knee and watched him race away. I would never see him again. A friend of his in tow stopped and stared. I got up, shaken. "What's his problem?" His pal mustered a "Sorry" and rode off.

I was picked on as a kid about as much as any other kid, I suppose. Maybe a little more—I was small. I got smacked around from time to time, but I would never say I had been bullied. But this incident I still remember. I was angry, frightened, and frustrated, and I wanted nothing more than to run that kid down with my sweet Mongoose. In fact, I remember distinctly that when I got home and found Mom, I burst into tears, wailing, "This is why I want to take kah-roddy!" Poor Mom. And so, I started training.

If I've learned one secret since, one that beats all others, it's that we have to stick around long enough to learn anything. But it takes a strong will to persevere through a process that is marked by uncertainty and false confidence, like martial training can be. Discipline is the only way through.

The main reason most people do not train, do not train consistently, or stop training is obvious—it's hard. It doesn't help that pop culture has written everything martial into a book so brazenly unrealistic it's unreadable. And commercialization too often turns training into a mass-market product, rather than reaffirming it as a life-enhancing process that tempers our ego.

Training is not straightforward, and is a frustrating journey depending on one's style, one's teacher, and how we perceive them. But such is the state of politics, education, religion, and name-your-philosophy. Like them, the martial path offers confusing, even contradictory, approaches to dealing with and solving life's practical matters, let alone afford usefulness for life-and-death confrontations.

Does this mean martial arts are not worth training in? Certainly and absolutely not. But I do think it means most people aren't clear about what training can actually provide them, and it shows in the number of folks who are training long term—not many. See, it's not the beginning that's hard—lots of people try martial arts—it's the staying that is. Most who begin training will not stay; they'll leave, to be replaced by newer students.

A few years ago, a martial arts school owners' periodical reported that 85 percent of those studying martial arts in America are thirteen years old or younger. I'll buy that.

Here's me interpreting the rest:

- A majority of that leftover 15 percent, say, 10 percent, is between the ages of thirteen and twenty-one.
- The remaining 5 percent is composed of us "twenty-one-and-olders."
- The majority of that 5 percent—up to 4 percent—is made up almost exclusively of new students who are beginning and others

who are leaving, training anywhere from three months to twenty years.

- That leaves just 1 percent of folks older than twenty-one who are engaged in martial training for more than twenty years.
- And my last bet: less than half of that 1 percent will train in martial arts as a life pursuit.

In fact, it's probably not even that high—very few people study throughout their lives. Break the numbers down however you like, compared to the population, the result is teensy.

Temperance in the form of discipline to stick around and keep training is not simply achieved through our force of will. A strong will can attempt even ludicrous feats—Evel Knievel strapped himself to a rocket, for God's sake, and even then could not successfully jump the Snake River valley. Our staying power has a lot to do with *why* we're training in the first place.

Now, "why" may seem like an easy question to answer since everybody's got an answer, but are those answers good enough to push back against the percentages and keep us training? In most cases, there are a host of other ways one can attain similar outcomes without so many punches to the face.

Self-confidence. It may take years, decades in some cases, for students to even begin to feel some presence of ability. This has to do with the art one is learning, its teaching methods, and the presence or absence of a student's acumen. The process of educating students has always been an issue of strong debate. Is *kata* (form practice) the beginning and end of training, or is it sparring, or a combination of the two, or neither? Should a student simply be drilled to react with preprogrammed responses? Or is the essence of ability infusing the moment with spontaneous creativity? And if it is, how does one achieve that? In the end, confidence can be fleeting and merely borrowed from others within the dojo.

If confidence is what you seek, then become a teacher, a mentor, or a "big brother." Take responsibility for the welfare and knowledge of another, perhaps someone younger or less fortunate than you. In the meantime, clean yourself up. More often than not, we know exactly what's wrong with us. If we picture ourselves as we'd like others to see us, we can study, learn, and live up to those standards. We can lose weight or become more successful, nicer, or better looking. Find people who exemplify the qualities you would like to have and hang around them. Want to be a nicer person? Hang out with people nicer than you.

Spiritual refinement. Can martial training refine one's spirit? Sure. Maybe. I guess. It depends on what you mean. Many are not clear as to how or why refinement occurs. Better to volunteer your time to those less fortunate than you. This is the best way to activate your compassion, kindness, and leadership to become someone of refined or "illuminated" spirit. Religion can offer spiritual guidance. Perhaps choose one, become more involved in your current one, or return to your faith, study it, and follow it more deeply.

Health and fitness. Can martial arts keep you fit? It can. But fitness is not the goal of martial training; it is ancillary to it. If you really want to get fit, join a gym and spend your money on a personal trainer.

Competition. Competitive martial arts are nothing new—judo became an Olympic sport in 1964—but their mainstream acceptance is. Thanks to events such as the Ultimate Fighting Championship, mixed martial arts (MMA) has become a force. And, like any sport, its main emphasis is on power, speed, and strength—the bigger, stronger, and faster one is, the better one's chances of victory. But in terms of martial arts, this is simply unsustainable—we don't get stronger, faster, and more power-ful as we age. I also see MMA culture too often characterized by over-confident, smug attitudes carefully crafted by PR experts for maximum payout at events but unhealthy in character, let alone for children who wish to emulate "hero" fighters.

And I have to laugh anytime I hear someone touting MMA as "real" fighting for self-protection. It's usually something about how all fights "go to the ground," or that it's "no holds barred." MMA is a sport, played in a ring against one other person, in a controlled and sterile environment, with time limits, referees, doctors, security, rules, regulations, insurance, and the training reflects that.

If anything, MMA is for short-term gain, certainly not long term, for there are examples of mature fighters, "legendary," even, losing in the ring, beaten by younger and less experienced fighters. This doesn't show the supremacy of MMA; it only highlights the deficiencies in relying on physical might. Better to join a local sports league for friendly competition and stop worrying about all those kicks to the head.

Self-defense. This is the biggie, the main reason I hear from folks interested in training. But useful self-defense skills, plus the awareness to use them, take years to habituate, and they are most often acquired through the marketplace, where many instructors maintain a sports mentality. This can often lead to rough training based on the application of power and speed. And, what's worse, rely on strategies like attacking the attacker—an awfully precarious decision because switching roles with an attacker is super-duper dangerous. If given a choice, who would actually wish their loved ones to train to confront or subdue violence, rather than simply resist and escape it? I wouldn't want my wife or children training to "beat up" their attacker, and they certainly don't want me doing it either. Naïveté kills.

Everyday life, provided it is reasonably safe and secure, has a knack for allaying our own sense of primal fear about defending ourselves from violence. This is human nature expressing itself—we tend to take for granted the things we come to expect, such as security, trust, health, and even the bounty of our lives. Instead of self-defense, join a gym and keep yourself in great shape. Running away is mankind's oldest form of self-defense. Keep a cell phone handy, one with GPS enabled, so others can locate you, and critically look at the vulnerabilities of your life. If you wanted to attack you, how would you do it? Shore up and close off those openings by layering your personal security through the lenses of location, lifestyle, and activity. The question to answer is essentially this: Are your choices and behavior leading you toward greater vulnerability? If you don't trust yourself to answer accurately, ask those whom you do trust for their honest thoughts.

The truth for the majority of people who decide to train is that martial arts will only ever be a pop-culture hobby, a semi-mysterious pastime to engage in when they are not busy working out or bar hopping. Westerners are immigrants to Eastern martial arts. Since landing on our shores, we have tried hard to define them for ourselves, and in doing so we've had to translate a foreign cultural identity. No easy feat. For better *and* worse, pop culture has largely done the work for us—I got hooked on Lee Van Cleef's ninja-themed TV show, *The Master*, in sixth grade, and I can still sing the theme song.

Is it any wonder there are tremendous misconceptions about martial arts and their seemingly mystical properties? In fact, under American law there is no basic formula for the application of unarmed self-defense, and in some cases a person's training might actually be used against them legally, even if they are incompetent or new to training.

There will always be a concern about racing past underlying philosophy, whitewashing it, or, worse, taking it for granted. The risk is building a house on sand—it's good to articulate answers. But answers get pretty complex when defining training's aspects, even basics. In fact, I can't think of any aspect of the martial way that doesn't relate to its whole—universals are like that. Imagine trying to describe the "what" or "how" of one strand of a spider's web without explaining the entire web itself, the spider that weaves it, and why it must do so.

"Why" questions are normally the hardest to answer, for they seek to clarify reason and purpose. But they also try to make sense of something deeper and more intrinsic to human nature: motive. Motive is at the heart of reason and purpose, and all values stem from it. In learning to become part of the ageless story of the martial way, we are bound to the intrinsic responsibility of learning to use its knowledge ethically or risk repeating the mistakes of history.

For me, training is a self-and-others value—we begin for ourselves, but ultimately we must balance it for the sake of others by teaching, coaching, and providing the best opportunity to extend the martial way's message of protecting and defending life. In fact, I like to think I don't even teach martial artists—I train protectors.

How can we ever live up to this auspicious, noble thought if we are confused about the spirit of our own martial nature? And the only way to truly understand that nature is to remain a *disciplined* student of it.

There's a great saying to become familiar with: *Gambatte!* Japanese for "Keep going!" Inevitably, someone will ask a worthwhile question during training and receive it as an answer. It's an interesting answer, as it manages to both encapsulate the spirit of the martial way and feel like someone just conned you out of ten bucks.

If there is a secret to martial arts and its training, it is found in this little phrase regarding constancy, longevity, and, most of all, discipline, since integrity as a virtue is nothing without the discipline to attain and maintain it. The saying itself may seem trite, and it's easy to understand why: if I were lost and asked a local for directions and he said, "Keep going!" with a big grin, I probably wouldn't grin back; I'd drop a safe on his head. "Keep going!" is one of those nonanswer answers. Very Zen. Zen's not a bad answer, mind you, except if you're drowning and would rather have a life preserver than a one-hand-clapping koan.

If patience is a virtue, then perseverance and its discipline are divine. But this kind of clarity takes time. And even when we think we're certain of that clarity, it can still remain elusive. Don't believe me? Try this: Imagine you are given the chance to travel back in time and meet yourself before beginning training or some other long-standing expertise. What expert advice would you give yourself regarding it?

Now, granted, there may be folks out there who could think of something specific. But for the majority of folks (and everyone I have ever asked this question of), their answer is nothing less than a big smile and a shaking of the head—no idea (my wife said, "It's all good," only reinforcing my point). I mean, what could you say?

The moment with yourself is a paradox, for even though you recognize all that is in store, all of the triumphs and failures, the good and the bad, there is no specific answer we can articulate that can fully justify a conclusion because beginner you is not ready to appreciate that significance. So, we're left with a new truth: take the journey, because it's a journey worth taking—discovery is in the exploration itself, not the destination.

So, how does one possibly encapsulate years of training and experience and distill them into a single thought?

"Keep going!"

It is frustrating in its simplicity because what we expect is not what we find. I mean, how can a secret be a secret when everyone already knows it? Easy—when they cannot perceive its intrinsic value. The writer G. K. Chesterton said, "An adventure is only an inconvenience rightly considered." Martial training is the adventure of adversity. And, like all of the universal aspects of the martial way, mastery lies as much in the command of that duality as it does in the surrender to it. But only the journey itself—a constant, disciplined quest—can strengthen our capacity to perceive its good.

Context Counts

Instead of turning ethical scenarios into twisted riddles, what's needed is clarity of action. Everyone deserves to be rescued, but logistically and tactically, it's a difficult feat. As people trained to risk themselves and protect others, lifeguards and martial artists are in a unique position to attempt those risky logistics and tactics to protect everyone, to the limit of their own ability.

Of course, lifeguarding a beach is not the same as dealing with a crazed attacker. Engaging in justifiable violence is like any cultivated trait: it must be habituated to become a working response. No one really expects people to pit themselves against a bloodthirsty killer, but that doesn't mean the morally correct answer is always to do nothing.

The Internet rightly blew up over the brutal murder of Kevin Joseph Sutherland on that DC Metro line. The passengers who witnessed the attack, huddled in the fore and aft of the car, gave accounts that were fraught with fear, confusion, and self-doubt. "You're not really sure what you need to do. . . . This man is holding a bloody knife. I don't think anyone was going to try and stop him," said a fifty-two-year-old woman who chose to remain anonymous.[4] Another claimed to have been present when Sutherland died but did not regret his inaction, stating, "What I don't wish is that I had somehow tried to attack the assailant. I am a little bit larger than he was, but I would not have won. It's scary, because if we had been sitting closer and had seen the attack start I probably would have tried to help, and would have been stabbed."[5] Since no one in that train car, about ten other souls, physically intervened to defend Sutherland, it predictably led folks to denounce or applaud the inaction.

Is it morally wrong not to intervene to save another's life when it is under brutal attack? In the real world, the answer is not simply yes or no, it's "It depends." And it depends on, at the very least, two contextual factors: one's physical capacity for such action and the circumstances.

Intervention is always weighed against one's physical capacity for such action. Say someone falls overboard and you're certain that leaping into the water is a death sentence because you can't swim. It's not morally wrong not to leap in. *But do something*. Throw a life jacket, alert authorities—the person's life is in your hands. Perhaps if one is an expert swimmer the answer *might* be different—"might" because individuals should still weigh their chances of success against those of condemning themselves. However, if an individual armed with a firearm is witness to that train attack and chooses not to intervene, it is grossly immoral.

The second aspect deals with the circumstances: those waters might not seem so deep if it's a baby that's drowning, especially if it's your baby. We may just throttle any attacker, whether they are armed or unarmed, and whether we are trained or untrained, if the attacker is killing an innocent, especially if it's our innocent.

If you're unwilling to risk harm or death to protect a complete stranger, that doesn't make you weird, it makes you human. Is it perhaps, then, just as moral a decision for normal folks not to intervene and instead choose to protect themselves?

No.

The decision not to intervene and instead protect oneself does not hold equivalent moral weight, though it may be a permissible act. The untrained majority has a far higher chance of succumbing to violence when intervening, which is why they generally choose not to. Had Sutherland's attacker not had a knife and only been beating him to death, the odds increase that others might have stepped up. Might. But the melee weapon was a game changer.

On some level many would like to believe that protecting ourselves is just as worthy as protecting others. "Don't be a hero!" may be an actual phrase, but what we correctly mean by it is that we should not take chances that *unnecessarily* risk our lives. And what is undoubtedly true, is that if we all abided by its literal meaning, in every context and circumstance, the world would be a much poorer place.

However, it is always moral should we choose to intervene in order to defend another's life by risking our own. Knowing this, we ought not revel in selfish isolationism and certainly not finger wag others into dispassionate inaction simply to justify our abstention.

What we can assure ourselves with is that the more training we have and the better skilled we are, the better our chances of protecting others in need. Thus, what is needed is the one thing that separates the novice from the expert, the layman from the initiated—*training*.

Without training, we are absent a crucial element for overcoming adversity and conflict—the physical models of willful self-risk.

For example, let's say you're enjoying an evening out with your significant other. Upon exiting a restaurant, you are greeted by a brawling crowd in the parking lot.

What should you do?

A. Retreat to the safety of the restaurant and call authorities.

B. Resist attacks from the group as you escape the area.

C. Extract the person most at risk.

D. Intercede and stop the fighting.

E. Confront those that pose a danger to others.

F. Subdue perpetrators.

The truth is that *any* of these options may be the right thing to do—it all depends on the context. If it's your significant other who is about to be set upon by the crowd, you may very well enter the fray. If it's your family or friends who are brawling, you may intercede and separate everyone. If police officers are about to be overwhelmed, you may decide to go to their aid by confronting aggressors. If you are law enforcement, you may have to subdue those involved and arrest them. Bear in mind, each of these options may be completely appropriate even if you know no one involved but simply recognize when strangers are in need of protection and defense.

Knowing the ethical context informs us of what we ought to do and then indicates the tactical action we *can* take based on our level of ability. Should we escape, defend ourselves, or protect others? Once we reconcile our ability with the situation through its context, we can then judge and take the prudent action. If you've a high level of skill but you're sick or injured, then escaping and regrouping is for you. If you're low skilled but a loved one is under attack, it would be hard not to intercede.

I count six ethical contexts for martial endeavor, listed hierarchically from lowest to highest in terms of difficulty:

1. Escape
2. Resist
3. Extract
4. Intercede
5. Confront
6. Subdue

To **escape** is to reposition in order to protect oneself from immediate danger, threat, and conflict: running away, outmaneuvering, seeking cover or concealment, driving off, whatever. In these cases, escaping ends the conflict. To embrace the protector ethic, escape must always be the first level of martial training that everyone learns and understands, especially kids. In physical training, escape takes the form of the dynamic body in action, which develops familiarity with landing and rebounding from the ground, and preventing injury. This may involve tumbling and leaping skills, climbing, and vaulting. If students cannot attain skill enough to physically reposition and maneuver themselves away from danger in the vein of escape so they can regroup and reassess to reduce or eliminate any imminent threat, no other training will matter.

To **resist** is what we typically think of as self-defense. When escape is not an immediately available option, we resist until we can facilitate an escape. This will involve times when one is trapped or physically caught and cannot get away. Resisting means removing oneself from another's grip—whether that's a bear hug or a wrist, lapel, elbow, or hair grab—or a tackling or mounted position, even defeating restraints such as rope, duct tape, handcuffs, or flex ties. It also involves recognizing the range of the body's natural weapons: the variety of fist and hand positions, elbows, knees, legs, feet, and even the teeth and head, not to mention the best and most reliable weapon of all, the body's full weight. One should also be familiar with the body's targeted points of weakness: the eyes and throat, soft spots of the head and face, nose, teeth, groin, anus, and armpits. There are a number of weak points or "pressure points" that riddle the body, but their utilization takes study and experience.

To **extract** is to go to the aid of others, specifically to extricate and evacuate them to reduce or prohibit threat and undue harm. These are people who may be injured or simply require evacuation from an area. Under the stress of a dangerous situation, one may become confused as to the action to take. In these cases, choose to extract someone else, as a bodyguard might, and make that person's protection and defense your job—saving yourself by saving others.

To **intercede** is to go to the defense of others. It's to lend resistance in their stead so they can safely escape or you can extract them. The challenge here is in remembering that this action is about defending them, with the goal of escape or extraction. There are times when well-intentioned folks go to the aid of others in conflict, only to throw matches on gasoline because they attack the attacker. Escalation in threats or violence might not end well and in the meantime increases the peril of those trapped by it, not to mention bystanders, and the one interceding. It even puts an enemy at greater risk, as escalation may be met with broader resistance and violence that may force one's hand to turn deadly.

To **confront** is to attack an enemy, whether openly or through deception. It may be considered necessary when preventing someone from entering your secure area, be it your home or anywhere else that must be defended. The range of tactics here involve all kinds of aspects; however, they are best trained by naturalizing movements so as to obscure their application in ambiguity and thereby ambush opponents to grant them little to no time for response. This involves a great deal of training—years—which is why *confront* sits near the top of this hierarchy.

To **subdue** is to effect the submission of threats through the incapacitation or physical confinement of an individual by joint locks, pain compliance, holds, or physical restraints that halt further confrontation. This is by far the most difficult aspect to achieve, for it calls to the highest order of ability and sheer will: sparing (and ultimately protecting) the enemy's life.

A lot of martial training concentrates on the practice of techniques by rote memorization so that muscle memory can form and the movements can then simply occur, even without conscious thought, when needed. At least, that's the tale we buy into. Personally, I don't even like it when I accidentally swear when I'm trying hard not to, so I am not a fan of a methodology for my body to react without my consent. "My body just reacted" is an especially unpleasant court defense, as juries tend not to appreciate thoughtless beatdowns from Sensei Kick-'Em-All.

Technique-oriented focus is useful when introducing and familiarizing students with traditional or highly technical movements. The danger is in reliance on it. Learning techniques as answers inevitably drives the moment of their use—if one has a hammer, everything else is generally a nail. This is not only naïve, it can be deadly to the user who forces a technique on an unwilling subject in a threatening situation. Lousy martial artists are like lousy magicians here—obvious and oblivious to it.

The protector ethic compels us to embrace tactics of unlimited creativity. This is simple logic: if we can never be certain as to what exactly we will encounter in terms of opposing variables, then the broadest method of extemporaneous defense ought to be embraced. Thus, turning our attention toward the *ethical context* first can broaden our awareness of technical options under those given conditions no matter which art we're training in.

The short of it: we must know techniques, but as their practitioner we are ultimately responsible for their choice, application, and consequences. This is a commonality all martial artists share regardless of style. The techniques chosen will vary, but their ethical usage is something everyone must aspire to.

The Hero and the Warrior

My favorite quote from the movie *Skyfall* occurs when secret agent James Bond meets his new quartermaster, Q, the designer of his spy tech and furrowed brow to many of his boyish antics:

"I'll hazard I can do more damage on my laptop sitting in my pajamas before my first cup of Earl Grey than you can do in a year in the field," quips Q.

"Oh, so why do you need me?" Bond replies.

"Every now and then a trigger has to be pulled," Q states.

Bond smiles. "Or not pulled. It's hard to know which in your pajamas."

Bond is talking ethics here, and it's about as ethical as the secret agent has ever sounded. As he rightly points out, the most important aspect is not simply the time, space, and opportunity for the weapon but also the ethical awareness of whether we ought to fire. Our ethic is both a natural and necessary part in our identification of choices and should be ever present in the pursuit of warriorship.

But search "warriorship" online and you'll be bombarded by spirit animals, sales of crystals, and archaic iconography, as it's bandied about in New Age circles. Warrior coaching, self-mastery, and finding the "inner warrior" are all just clever marketing schemes. No one seems to understand how to even define warriors, let alone train others in their ways. So why invoke the warrior at all? Because we associate the archetype with an ideal: the centered, unflappable person able to protect and defend against life's challenges for self and others. In that sense, a warrior is really a hero.

Yet the warrior goes beyond what heroes are capable of. Warriorship is not a complicated thing, but it's certainly not easy. Its roots are associated with war and conflict, to be sure, but not confined or limited to it. The best definition I ever heard of a warrior came from Jack Hoban, in an interview I did with him several years ago:

A fireman is a hero. He protects life, right? At the risk of his own life. Runs into a burning building to protect someone he's never seen before. Perhaps as a volunteer. And could die saving this person he doesn't even know. That's a hero. That's the epitome of the self and others [value]. Which others? All others.

And what does he get for it? If he's a volunteer he doesn't get anything material. If he works for a town maybe he gets a civil servant's pay. But what he [does] get for it is two things: one, he gets to save lives, which is the most noble, best feeling that a human being can get, and he gets the esteem and support of his peers and the people that he saved. He gets the inner and the outer feeling.

So, what's the difference between them and a warrior? A warrior is supposed to protect people at the risk of his own life, but what he does that [others do not] is *kill* to protect life; this oxymoronic thing that actually undermines this feeling of nobility from defending others.

Yes, I did protect others. Yes, I did protect life, but I had to take life in order to do it. This is an added burden. They almost cancel each other out. And that's why people get sick from it. And they'll surely get sick if they do it from the wrong mental perspective, out of anger or fear or prejudice or disrespect or dehumanization—you'll get real sick. But even if you don't, it's very, very difficult.

And that's why a warrior to me is the epitome of human endeavor because even though they protect life they may have to take it which is almost, so dangerous to you, that it can't be overlooked.[6]

There's a burden and responsibility here. Is it right to be excited by the pomp and circumstance of martial training, the scope of its history, the minutiae and relentless pursuit of technical mastery? Sure. This is the "self" side, the selfish part we often, perhaps too often, get energized about because it's what we can most easily and readily identify with. But we should be mindful not to allow ourselves to be carried away by the best intentions of our enthusiasm, lest it devolve into pride and self-centeredness.

There is an "others" side to training as well, steeped in the honesty of movement, viable usage of space, and the ethics of the protector. We channel it through the principles of training, which gives us the macro view that provides the necessary counterweight to find the stability to reconcile the two halves. It is our mature side, the adult in us, providing perspective to be real about our movement and come to terms with its inherent burden and accept it. We accomplish this through self-risk: mixing ourselves and our capabilities into any set of choices that we can rationally identify.

Here's a true story for you. When marines went house to house in Fallujah, looking for insurgents at the height of the Iraq War, it was a terrible and costly business. Tactics included tossing flash-bang grenades into suspect houses before storming in. On this particular occasion, a young marine leading point on his team approached a door, grenade in hand, and reached for the handle. But before he had even touched it, it swung open, and standing there, AK-47 in hand, was an insurgent, with more milling in the room behind him. The young marine looked at the insurgent, and the insurgent looked at the marine. And then, casually, the marine offered him the grenade. The insurgent took it and the marine closed the door. Do I really have to write *BOOM*?

The actions this young man took to position, leverage, and initiate options in his area of operation are indicative of the raw fundamentals of the martial way. And it's safe to say he was never trained to hand a live grenade to an insurgent. But when he came face to face with his enemy, a veil was pulled over those options, confusing an otherwise relentless adversary into voluntarily accepting a grenade with his own hands. Does that mean it's a legitimate technique? People confused about truth, which is sometimes illogical and unreasonable, and instead relying only on prepatterned occurrence are going to have trouble here. I can just picture marines drilling this "technique" and yelling—because I always picture marines yelling like R. Lee Ermey—WHEN YOU APPROACH THE DOOR, HAVE YOUR GRENADE IN HAND! WHEN THE INSURGENT OPENS THE DOOR, YOU WILL HAND HIM THE GRENADE!

The moral in this example lies not in exactly what the marine did but in why the marine did what he did—to protect other marines. Anyone else in that scenario might have gotten themselves shot or killed, or started a firefight that endangered civilians and teammates. The lesson is don't lose your head under stress, and train hard and well so you don't. There's the truth. If it's a fancy new technique you're looking for, start with that one. Not only is it logical, it's totally reasonable.

Training isn't just about learning to use martial arts more effectively. It's also about recognizing that we are more effective through consistent training. It is this thought that must come first. For if it does not, then waiting to be instructed is all about training to become good at some point in the future, instead of training to be good today.

Learning to fight or defend only yourself is a selfish, immature act in the long run. The better way is to see training as a conduit to becoming the kind of person we wish ourselves to be—a protector, teacher, leader— the kind of person who is in control and command when there is conflict, even violence. The kind of person others seek out when they need help.

Not just a hero but a warrior.

Integrity

Of my high school memories, there is Ben, a jock and all-around cool kid, playing the heavy in the locker room after gym class—he was half-joking, but only half. Imitating the high kicks he undoubtedly saw on *Samurai Sunday*, a weekly kung fu feast on our local channel 66, he threw awkward roundhouses at me, a back kick at others. Bobby, a quintessential pencil-necked geek who came back from summer break having found an extra foot in height and another fifty pounds to block for the football team, quipped about a little information being a dangerous thing. As if to prove him wrong, Ben swung a lopsided, back-spinning Dunning-Kruger that accidentally hit Bobby. There was a lot of yelling after that amid Ben's profuse "sorrysorrysorry."

The poet Alexander Pope nails it:

> A little learning is a dang'rous thing;
> Drink deep, or taste not the Pierian spring:
> There shallow draughts intoxicate the brain,
> And drinking largely sobers us again.

The unfortunate story out of Raleigh, North Carolina, in July 2015, is a grim reminder of Pope's insight. Tracy Williams was murdered in the middle of the afternoon in a Food Lion parking lot by her estranged boyfriend. The tragedy was made worse by the fact that it might not have been so tragic. Williams had armed herself with not one but two firearms, the training to use them, and a permit to carry. She was ready, or so she hoped. She even switched up the car she'd been driving to obscure her trail from her wannabe lover, a man she asked courts twice to issue restraining orders against.

When finally ambushed, Williams drew down, fired, and hit her attacker in the leg, slowing but not stopping him. After her first shot, her gun jammed. She had a second gun, which she did not draw. She did not draw it because, according to reports, she screamed for help and tried to escape, giving her enemy critical time to load his own gun, run her down, and execute her. He was later arrested by a SWAT team and charged with first-degree murder.

I do not write this to criticize Williams; that would be unfair. She has my deepest respect, for she did far more and acted more bravely than many would have under the same circumstances. She perceived a real threat and invested in her defense. Rather than move away and forge a new life, she took a stand for the one she had built and even defended it from her very own archenemy. She got herself trained, purchased firearms, legalized herself to carry, and did. But the moment, like any moment might for anyone trained, overwhelmed and consumed her. Make no mistake, Williams died fighting for her life, and she deserves our admiration and respect. Her tragic outcome would be all the worse if we did not take some lesson from it: to drink deep of the Pierian spring *and keep drinking*.

There's a saying, "You will fight the way you train." And it's true. If our training relies on intense, high-stress, fear-inducing clashes between partners, and afterward we are emotionally spent, then we are most probably training ourselves to intuit and reenact all of these same experiences during actual confrontation. We may think we're arming ourselves by engaging with these experiences regularly to "inoculate" us to their impact, when in actuality they might just be blunting our effectiveness by making us just a little sick each session.

There's a trend in training that is summed up basically as "out-thug the thug." It's a strategy in which an attack is met by an even attackier defense, and, after a moment, one looks just like the other. It reminds me of comedian Mike Myers, who coined the Scottish martial art "Fa-Que!" He said it's "mostly just head butting and then kicking people when they're on the ground."

We're only ever as mighty as our next opponent because chances are we'll actually be at some disadvantage, be it that we're weaker than they are, or injured, or surprised. And then Popeye-ing open that can of spinach so we can "thug" others, who are in the process of "thugging" us, gets right messy. When training becomes too myopic, it can strip out the techniques that some might find impractical, like high kicks or something. But it can also strip the character-building stuff. So, if your answer to every conflict is "Fa-Que!" and a head butt, check to see if you're Mike Myers. If not, you might want to reassess your training.

The heart of the issue is this: if, to overcome hard, fast, and aggressive violence, we ourselves are forced to action that is even harder, faster, and more aggressively violent, we're on a slippery slope. The real problem with "out-thugging the thug" is not its working; it's that it isn't *worth* working. To out-thug, there's a good chance we'll have to habituate our behavior and train to act thuggish and become that which we despise. No thanks. Marvel Comics fans don't condemn Bruce Banner for not perpetually living life as the unstoppable Hulk because we recognize that living as an ever-paranoid beast who trusts no one is an unhappy, soul-sucking way to live. When everyone is viewed as a potential enemy, everyone gets treated as one, and you can include friends and loved ones on that list.

Training does not have to be some perpetual roller coaster of stress inoculation. Learning to become a good defensive driver does not entail constantly smashing into other cars so we can handle an accident. It means habituating one's driving habits and awareness so as to have the time and space to respond effectively to emergencies regardless of the conditions. This is not a perfect analogy, but I think it a far tastier recipe than brutalizing ourselves and others in regular training just to gain what we think is some modicum of advantage.

Now, for dangerous jobs, such as serving warrants and military operations, consistent, high-stress training can be beneficial for those specific high-stress moments because it trains one in known operational tactics reflexively, so they can become second nature. But in those cases, operators generally know, even dictate, those moments of conflict in advance, as well as who their enemy is, what they are capable of, and under what context and conditions they will be faced. Success in those operations is most often shaped by operators' proactiveness.

But the rest of us do not have the luxury of prescient intel about what kind of spontaneous conflict or violence we may face in the daily course of our lives, let alone from exactly whom. Most folks train in martial arts simply because they like it, and maybe they want to learn how to be a better person for their little part of the world. Thus, training does not require us to rely on access to the X-Men's Danger Room or put ourselves through the gauntlet of Sakura's ninja Octagon right behind Chuck Norris. (I say "rely" here because some danger rooming and Octagoning is often a lot of fun in context.)

Life is difficult, stressful, and scary enough on its own to provide us with all the itinerant changes and variable conditions that we can possibly handle. These conditions will be such that we'll be forced to deal with them in ways that'll make our responses far more difficult to determine than we could possibly imagine or anticipate in any regular training session. And as we are the ones who have chosen to risk ourselves, we must choose: How do we wish to respond to conflict? With pent-up anxiety and stress? Or cool and collected? I'm not saying that just by believing ourselves to be calm and cool, we will be. It isn't that simple. We have to train and habituate ourselves physically and meta-physically until we actually are. Marinating ourselves in invented stress, anxiety, and fear may only multiply those aspects under real-world conditions.

There is nothing to suggest that a "well-rounded training" ideal and the "highly competent protector" ideal are mutually exclusive. In my world they are not; in fact, the more competent one is and the higher one's ability, the more one can gain the confidence to reach goals regarding character and virtue.

We should train ourselves the way we wish to live, lead, and fight—calmly and collectedly. That means enjoying training, laughing, having a good time, protecting your partners, telling a joke. Be inspired and look forward to training. And, when finished, we should feel better (and better in ability) for having done it.

Nothing ensures that physical training will be there to make the difference for us. We do not train to simply prepare ourselves for conflict—civilians are not law enforcement or the military—but rather to face up to the truth of who it is we aim to be. This means we aren't training simply to sharpen up a few skills or perform a bunch of formulistic techniques—it is immature to think so. We are training for a far more important reason: to make better ethical decisions. And to do so, we have to risk ourselves in our moral reasoning so we can identify better choices. No easy feat, since to do so involves changing the person we are and living up to who we know we ought to be.

Only our personal integrity can authorize us as warriors and protectors to accomplish this.

NOTES

1. Raymond Nickerson, "Confirmation Bias: A Ubiquitous Phenomenon in Many Guises," *Review of General Psychology* 2, no. 2 (June 1998): 175.
2. Elizabeth Ashford and Tim Mulgan, "Contractualism," in *The Stanford Encyclopedia of Philosophy*, fall 2012 ed., ed. Edward N. Zalta, https://plato.stanford.edu/archives/fall2012/entries/contractualism/.

3. For those who dislike changes to their ethical riddles, I say this: the reason ethical questions are composed in the first place is to allow one to think them out. If right and wrong are only to be determined by one's gut in knee-jerk fashion, this denies us any opportunity to explore the process and discern new options and, hence, new perceptions.

4. Peter Hermann, Michael Smith, and Keith L. Alexander, "Horrified Passengers Witnessed Brutal July 4 Slaying Aboard Metro Car," *The Washington Post*, July 7, 2015, accessed October 23, 2017, https://www.washingtonpost .com/local/crime/victim-in-metro-slaying-stabbed-repeatedly-during -robbery-on-train/2015/07/07/8dd09132-249b-11e5-b72c-2b7d516e1e0e _story.html?utm_term=.5f3ebe229fe5.

5. "Horrific Details in the Murder of AU Grad, Kevin Sutherland, released. :(• r/washingtondc," Reddit, accessed October 23, 2017, https://www.reddit .com/r/washingtondc/comments/3cfp1p/horrific_details_in_the_murder_of _au_grad_kevin/csv6qx5/?context=10000.

6. Jack Hoban, "Ethical Warrior," Telephone interview by author, July 2010.

3

To Judge: Prudence as Vigilance

Wisdom from Knowledge

She was desperate. And the look she gave me was equal parts incredulous and I-will-so-murder-you-for-this-later. She pressed her boyfriend's face into her chest, shielding him from the brunt of a beatdown from his rivals during an ambush outside the student union. I did nothing, but watched the show.

In 1993, I was at the University of Illinois working my way through an undergraduate degree in philosophy. I did this so I could think deep thoughts about being unemployed. Philosophy students will find that funny; the world used to hinge on philosophy. In many cases it still does, thankfully, only now it's like that old joke no one is seriously telling anymore: seekers of truth find it hilarious, everyone else refuses to laugh.

On this night, I was working security for a party at which these rivals were stalking their prey. I'd been warned about them—gang members who'd traveled the two and half hours from Chicago to our little college town of Urbana. When I sized them up at the party, I was unimpressed. But when the party ended and they left, I admit, I was relieved.

And then I walked outside into a fight. At which point, I stopped and I watched. I did not intervene.

Inaction probably had something to do with the girl—a bestie of my recent ex-girlfriend. The breakup was a shock and the wound was fresh. I missed her. Maybe I wanted to exact grief on somebody who I thought had colluded to get me fired. Or maybe it was just the fact that I didn't want to defend a fool from other fools and risk becoming one myself. These screwballs were beneath me, I figured. Why risk myself for them? A friend who'd assisted me at the party looked for permission to mosh in that silly mosh pit, with an imploring, "Jimmy?" But having clocked out of my security duties, I answered him with a quizzical look, as in "No, stupid."

As soon as the bunch realized neither my friend nor I was going to engage them, they dug in and doled it out. Real gangs shoot you, or beat you with bats, or machete stab you, and now I know some beat a guy shielded by his girl. And then it was over. They retreated into the night, campus police arrived, the punching bag showed off his bloodied, swollen face, the girl glared at me, and I knew it was time to go. So I left.

But that moment has never left me. Her stare, and everything it stood for, was hot enough to brand. And it did.

Not long after, one of the fellows I was training on campus with—John, a six-foot bodybuilding bruiser who weighed in at 225—related a story from the night before. Returning home after a law school class, he came upon two quarreling groups. These were not mathletes arguing over calculus; they were drunk and nobody was backing down from whatever there was to back down from. When they clinched, somebody pulled a pipe. And when that pipe came down on one fellow's noggin, there was John, to disarm and take control of it. Then, like an angry dad, he sent everyone to bed. As he left, he overheard the fellow whose brain he'd just preserved say, "That guy just saved my life."

My first reaction was admonishment—you could have been hurt! Yes, he admitted, he could have been, but he wasn't. In fact, he told me he had done what he had done because he was training with me. I found that confusing.

I was the teacher of this small campus martial arts group, but I'd never advocated risking your skin to save a bozo, let alone crashing a gang fight to save a bunch of them. So where John got this notion was a head scratcher—it certainly wasn't me. At that time in my life, I was looking out for myself. I figured everyone else should too.

I didn't realize it, but I was acting out every bad kung fu movie—lots of spin-kicks but no story. And without story, there's no meaning. I was missing my third act, in which the protagonist changes for the better. The omission is anathema to storytelling, as conflict is the immutable challenge to be surmounted and only the hero manages to do so. Smarts, toughness, skill, and even humor are the tools of the hero and warrior (like a signature fedora), who always do the right thing to save the day.

But my problem was deeper than that. I wasn't even sure how I could know what that right thing was. How I could ascertain the right from the wrong, the wise from everything else.

Wisdom comes when we can properly value, reason, and judge to act on knowledge ethically, the hallmark of prudence. And for warriors, vigilance is the steady use of prudence to protect the good. Clearly, if we're going to train in the martial way, we need to judge right from wrong—lives hang in the balance.

Discerning Priorities

Right and wrong is only attainable when we're honest about reality. And being honest about reality is only possible when we tell the difference between things. To tell the difference is to discern, and discerning allows us to prioritize. Without priorities, all things are even and equal. And when no one thing is more important, sacred, or ideal, then all things are given a chance to jockey to be such. And it gets confusing.

Yanagi Ryuken was a purported master of aikido. He bragged of his 200-0 "no holds barred" fighting record in an interview with the gossip rag *Tantei File* and said he'd accept any challenger at any time to prove his skill. He also made the fantastic claim that he could defend himself without touching attackers. Using only the power of his "internal energy," known as *ki*, he could literally upend and thrash his own students from across a room, like a Jedi reaching out with the Force, or a wizard reaching out with his powers, or a cult leader reaching out with his damaging psychological hold on his brainwashed flock.

Shortly after publication of the interview, he was challenged by a ring fighter, Tsuyoshi Iwakura, a man half his age. Ryuken, so confident in his abilities, accepted a $5,000 bet that he'd win. On November 26, 2006, at the Hokkaido Prefectural Sports Center in Sapporo, Japan, and before an audience of five hundred people, this experiment to rediscover if water is in fact wet was called for brutality after only forty-seven seconds due to multiple drubbings to the master's untouchable face. Afterward, and having lost several teeth, Ryuken refused to budge regarding his energy abilities, excusing his performance on his advanced age and the strength of his rival. He retired soon after with what he claimed was a 99 percent win rate.

Now, we could simply headline this "Fighter Loses Teeth, Blames Kicks," but there's a deeper lesson here. Ryuken was a product of his own confirmation bias. He continually confirmed the world he'd built around him and urged people who cared about him, from family to students, to keep confirming it by serving up false—untruthful— information.

When he decided to stop telling the difference between reality and his own twisted perception of it, he didn't just step back from the act of discriminating between differences. He absolved himself of the fact that there were differences at all. And he continued to do this, even after one of those differences kicked him in the mouth over and over.

The protector ethic is the DNA of the martial way. It is its most natural state because there would be no such thing as martial arts were it not for its ideal. But make no mistake, that DNA can be stripped out to make an open and empty vessel, like a stem cell, to ensconce any belief. When we don't clarify the good, or know how to, it disables us from making better decisions. Because when anything can be a priority—since no one thing is—training can be consumed not by the big stuff that's actually important but by the details of minutiae, or worse, something weird, like believing you have magic powers. Just speak with any battle reenactor, like a Civil War hobbyist, minutiae is far more important than efficacy of ability—they aren't actually going to refight Gettysburg, just make it look good. However, it may be true that warriors must fight for their lives or the lives of others. And if they must, it will also be true that in that moment the particulars of their training will not be as important as their raw ability under conditions. Efficacy trumps trivia.

Although Western fighting arts have their own storied history, as ancient as the Greeks, Eastern martial arts are rather new to the West, with interest in them beginning in the late nineteenth century. Pop culture would eventually get a stranglehold and squeeze until they turned blue, writing them into books, comics, TV, and movies. This benefited their proliferation, but it came with a price: inauthentic expectations that grew around the training like thorny weeds in a vegetable garden. Getting to the fruit was to risk getting stuck, or, worse, becoming so confused as to mistake the weeds for fruit and the fruit for weeds.

Priorities matter. We humans are not meant to roam compassless for the same reason our cell phones burn out earlier and faster when constantly locating a signal—our own human nature will defy us. If what we tell it to do is in reality innately unreasonable, we're easily confounded and place ourselves on the path to cynicism by our lack of direction, our misprioritization.

Martial training is an agent of change. If it weren't a method that provides confidence, awareness, physical defensive skills, or telekinesis (see what I did there?), folks simply would not volunteer for it. People train because they are convinced it will cause them to change in ways in which they are eager to change. There's great debate about what that change entails and even greater debate about how exactly to achieve it, but we can't deny the change itself. Like education or faith, when we participate voluntarily, martial training can transform our perception of the world. But if some believe this process is stalled, stopped, or, worse, does not exist, there's a good chance they may become disillusioned.

Disillusion is an interesting word. I've yet to find an actual definition, only similar words. *Disaffect. Disappoint. Dissatisfy.* When we are disillusioned with politics, it's due to politicians reneging and violating promises, and we're left deceived and betrayed. With religion, doubt can erode the belief there's an active God in people's lives, and a person of faith may come to believe there's no God at all. What they share in common is a loss of trust, which comes from uncertainty in discerning truth. And this is a precursor to accepting the idea that truth does not actually exist, except for whatever folks might decide is "true."

Applied to martial training, once we think truth is relative, everything becomes suspect, from style, to authorities, teachers, and ourselves—you can't even trust yourself. We wind up losing confidence in our ability to discern the necessary in training. And if there's no way to be certain about what's necessary, then truth *must* be relative—what's true for one is not true for another. And if *that's* the case, then maybe there's no such thing as truth at all and everything is just nonsense we tell ourselves about what we wish to believe.

Slipping into disillusionment is not about being unable to find what one is looking for—we'll always find something because humans tend to project importance on whatever it is we do find. *It's that we don't know what we ought to be looking for.* Try using a needleless compass. With no sense of direction, every route looks the same. Without a standard, such as magnetic north, how could we orient ourselves? And how could we sense truth?

"Conformity to fact or actuality; a statement proven to be or accepted as true,"[1] is what we find in the dictionary under *truth*. The takeaway is that assent is needed to "conform" and "accept." Facts are not truth. Facts represent actuality, but they only support, provide evidence, and can lead us to acceptance of truth.

As a tenet of the natural world, truth does not require consensus among people to exist. In fact, unanimity in the validity of truth only perpetuates the idea that it's malleable. Discernment of and fidelity to truth begs the question—it takes for granted that truth exists and can be discerned. "Truth is stranger than fiction," we accept, as it can be as unreal as lousy fiction, and just as unbelievable. Rediscovery then, is necessary, for certain undeniable issues are often taken for granted, or, worse, willfully ignored, even to the extent of lying to ourselves and others about their very existence.

The Painting or the Guard?

In my first year of graduate school for a master's in ethics, I took a class on "agency" and "action." This was theory discussing the nature of human willing, and yes, it was dry. Drinking a glass of sand was a waterslide of beer compared to this theory.

Of late, we were focusing on a modern philosopher. I didn't care for him, as he was ambiguous when it came to matters of right versus wrong. Now as then, for any philosopher to impress me, I like them to do this thing that most do not: take a crack at explaining *why* right is right and wrong is wrong. In other words, I like them to clarify their judgments.

There's nothing unusual about their omission, most common in the postmodern arena. You'll recall this "why" is known as the source of normativity: the reason, basis, motive, cause, aim, goal, purpose—none of these words is quite strong enough—for the sense of oughtness, obligation, of human behavior; the origin of why people choose to do what they do. These compelling feelings of obligation must come from somewhere, right? The long-standing philosophical question is, where exactly?

The reason for many philosophers' moral ambiguity is simple: they don't know. Or they're unwilling to take a stand about it. Even Aristotle in his *Nicomachean Ethics* never explained why right is right. He just said one needs a proper upbringing to understand ethics, which speaks to some intrinsic quality, one he never mentions. So, defining this why is an issue at least as old as the Greeks. The philosopher we were reading on this day had played mental Twister to expressly avoid explaining the why. And so we wound up discussing values, their nature, and how we find these values valuable.

Eventually the professor laid out in Sherlockian detail how the nature of "autonomy" was in essence to "decide for the self" just how values ought to be valued. "Not everything is about *ethics*," she said, the word a chore. "To some, there is great value in art. And when confronted with choices, reasonable questions on personal action are posed. What should we do? What should we not? Let us imagine a museum on fire. Amid the flames, we can either save only a priceless Van Gogh painting or wake up a sleeping guard. For the person of agency and action, this is a legitimately tough choice."

She looked to the faces of her students for approval.

Now, in comedy, there's a bit called the "spit take." You've probably seen it. A character does or says something odd, and a fellow character in the act of drinking reacts by spewing the contents. It is described thusly: "Reaction. One of surprise. The 'spit' action overly dramatized; a vehicle to convey shock or surprise humorously with an exaggerated visual."[2] Had I actually been drinking my glass of sand, it would have gone everywhere when she equated the value of a painting with the value of human life.

The student next to me went off: "What? That is a human being! A human life! How can you possibly compare the two?"[3] The professor straightened—a torrent of reasonableness at any university is a rare event and caught her off guard. Her response was, "Well, OK, if that's what you think."

It's hard to express just how I felt in the modern university experience. Most everyone I knew, from teachers, to classmates, to advisers, was utterly convinced of a particular reality to the world—that there can be no universal values, and, thus, no objective morals. Dissenters to this view, like myself, were often forced to covertly blend in like members of any fraternal organization working clandestinely for a lost cause.

Just imagine, for a moment, everyone you know believing that your daily dietary intake should consist of nothing more than roadkill. I'm not talking survival here, but regular calories consisting of animals in various states of decomposition. On its face you would be appalled at the notion in the midst of such bounty as our society produces. You would be compelled to challenge them as to why they would consider chowing on anything served up by the pavement, when just a few doors down there's a farmer's market, a grocery store, and a twenty-four-hour McDonald's with made-to-order french fries. On sale.

What you'd receive in response would be some ordered string of ten-dollar words, attributed to a philosopher who explained then, just as your friends must now explain to you, that eating roadkill is, without exception, very, very normal around the world. And yes, I agree, there can be no doubt that there are multitudes of people around the globe who eat all manner of beasts in all states of expiration, from fresh to just past oh-my-god-are-you-kidding-me? And there is also no doubt that these same folks have all kinds of reasons to do what they do. To them, in many unfortunate cases, it is a function of existence, because eating to exist is better than not eating, which invariably leads to not existing. And much of what my university friends would assure me with were examples of *how* all that sort of normalcy is utterly normal. But what they could not explain in plain, everyday language, is *why* it is universally normal.

And the trouble is that after eating so much roadkill, it not only affects the taste buds, it precludes most folks from clarifying and judging just what a decent meal really is. Since both can be eaten, in that restaurant from hell, roadkill is given the same status as roasted squab prepared by Jacques Pépin.

Why this is happening needs no study. It can be difficult to discern wisdom from knowledge. In other words, people mistake the one for the other. They mistake the knowing of something for the wisdom it may impart, as if existence is proof of efficacy. This suggests that all knowledge is wise, but it is actually the devaluation of wisdom.

Virtually, we have at our fingertips the vastness of human knowledge. With all that information at our disposal, it's no wonder many choose to treat it disposably. Our age of technology means it is spectacularly easy to embrace any kind of knowledge, even fraudulent or debunked, as original and wise. Thanks in part to this glut of information, truth must not just be discovered, it must be rediscovered, over and again. And it must be continually acknowledged as it competes with alternative thinking.

With that, let's take my professor's art versus life museum analogy to task:

The Museum Fire

You find yourself inside a museum that is on fire. Let us suppose you are the last person inside that you know of.

As you make your escape, you come to a fork in the hallway and can make out two distinct paths:

- One leads to a priceless, world-famous painting—your favorite—and would allow you to save it from certain destruction in your escape.
- The other leads to a snoring security guard, whom you could wake and escape with. The roar of the fire is enough to drown out any yell to wake the guard.

Which way should you go? There may not be time enough to take both actions and escape injury or death.

Do you have an obligation to protect and preserve the guard's life? You yourself are trying to escape, so we can discern that you at least value your own life. But let's put in a third option, one that might not be reasonable to everyone but may be at least justifiable from one's own perspective: wake the guard and tell him to skedaddle. Then, because you value "priceless" art, you can choose to risk your own life to rescue the painting as the building burns around you. This is not going to be reasonable to everyone, especially to people who love and care about you, but at least you're not risking the lives of others to satisfy your own personal concern and protect yourself to boot.

Perhaps to some the choice between saving the painting and saving the guard are equivalent. You might even have an argument for why saving the painting is a better choice than saving the guard. Except for this: when you are the guard. Or when the guard is someone you love and care about—a husband, father, brother, son, wife, mother, daughter, or sister. And here's the thing: chances are that guard is somebody's someone. The guard is somebody's father, daughter, whatever. And if you conclude it wouldn't be right for anyone to supersede the value of your own life or anyone you care about with their arbitrary values— such as fine works of art—then why would you believe it is in any way allowable for you to impose that on them?

My university professor was well respected and had recently played host to a symposium on world poverty and human rights with similarly minded people from around the globe. And yet there she was, in measured voice, rationally condemning a fellow human being to death because that person's life was simply outweighed by her own twisted sense of values. The same kind of twisting that allows dehumanization to take root—human life is not intrinsically valuable.

I really don't mind that she made the analogy—it was hypothetical, after all. And I like to think that under actual life-threatening circumstances, she would instinctively run down the hallway toward the snoring guard. Adrenaline-fueled calamities have a unique way of calibrating humans toward the protection of self and others. Just review the actions of regular folks during chaotic events—some people will risk their lives for others, whether during mass violence or natural disasters.

Now, if, in the face of all that, she *still* chooses the painting over the guard, then she's most likely part of that select group of folks known as sociopaths. Because let's face it, there is no argument that can justify choosing the painting over the life of an innocent person. If someone even tries, it indicates either willful ignorance or the belief that one's arbitrary concerns are worth more than other people's lives—a key aspect of sociopathy.

But for educational purposes, let's engage the argument from "autonomy" and "agency" to choose the painting over the guard with my professor. Here's what I would have said to her: So you have decided to rescue the painting. You run outside—saving yourself—and make it to the parking lot. You are looking up at the building, now engulfed in flames. A woman runs up to you—she's clutching two small children—and asks, "You were the last person to come out of the museum. My husband is a guard inside. Did you see him?"

Question: Would you tell her the truth or would you lie to her? And if you would lie, are you lying for her sake or are you lying for your own?

I say, you made your choice. You should stick by it and tell her the truth: you condemned her husband to die in order to save your favorite painting. You engaged your autonomy and agency to make that personal decision. Then hold the painting up and explain just how cool and famous it really is. Perhaps that will console her and her children over the loss of their husband, father, and provider now and in the future.

However, maybe you think you should lie to her. Maybe you feel you *have* to lie to her. But this raises another question: *Why would you feel that?* Is it because you don't want to hurt her feelings? Doubtful. Why would you care about her feelings? You certainly didn't care about the guard's, and you left him to die. If you are lying to her because you feel you have no choice and are forced to in that moment, then does that not clearly violate the prescriptive elements of independence and authenticity that autonomy and agency are defined to illustrate and you so vociferously defend?

But, of course, you could not tell her the truth. You would lie to her. And the why is simple: the lie is not for her, it's for you. It's to cover up the fact that you did something wrong, you know it, and you do not wish to reap the consequences. The lie is, in fact, because you're trying to protect, trying to preserve, your own life. Again. That's two saves in one day.

Know who could have used just one of those saves?

The guard.

Eye of the Beholder

Confused thinking prevents us from gaining ability in the martial way because we convince ourselves that the world is whatever we wish it to be, instead of seeing the world as it actually is. But it isn't just crazy people who engage in this. Most decent folks—including you, dear reader—are indoctrinated to think this way, and it comes from the most benign of places.

Although notions similar to the phrase "Beauty is in the eye of the beholder" have been around since the third century, the phrase did not catch on until the end of the nineteenth. Today it is the mantra of the modern artist. But far from providing any illuminating clarity, the expression epitomizes the ultimate state of aesthetic relativism and actually drains meaning from the word *beauty*. If beauty exists only in the opinion of its beholder, then there is no such thing as beauty or ugliness—how can they exist when only personal opinion and its preference are their definitional values?

Stop and think just how much this single notion has impacted the world. Its comfortable ambivalence permeates everything from morals, to how we view the elements of culture (ours and foreign), to our social, political, and religious institutions. Ambivalence is too often mistaken for thoughtfulness, making it appear intelligent and fashionable to resist judgments and come to no conclusions. Take this to its logical end: If you are an expert or considered such in any field, you are such no longer—how can any "expert" opinion exist, when all opinions matter equally? When we believe mere opining is enough to carry the burden of proof, art and its variants are just the distraught and wounded. But the blow to truth is fatal.

And here's the punch line: *beauty* and *ugly* mean exactly what they represent. Their etymologies relate to the enhancement of or detraction from life and its value, not mere personal preference or taste. *Beauty* is derived from the Greek *horaios*, meaning "hour" and applied to timeliness and ripeness, such as of fruit, perhaps to indicate optimal taste and nutritional value in food as medicine. The notion also applied to women in their prime—childbearing years. Even more telling is the definition of *ugly* as "morally offensive." There is nothing relativistic about these notions; they mean exactly what they are meant to mean. Beauty and ugliness exist in the world, and we have always been able to tell their difference. It's simply become fashionable to refrain.

From now on, try this expression as a far more precise one: *attractiveness is in the eye of the beholder*. Beauty notwithstanding.

We could make this clarification till the end of days, and yet the damage from this misguided notion has been done tenfold since the Enlightenment. It's a confusion that is especially present in the area of moral philosophy.

You'll recall that moral relativism is a theory championed by this past century's philosophy du jour, postmodernism, that essentially states that justifications for moral judgments are not universal but instead relative to the traditions, convictions, or practices of an individual or group. It's most often associated with the phrase "It's moral to me because I believe it is." It's as easy a theory to accept as a lottery payout. Cultures are different around the world, so why should we all share the same values and moral precepts? The concept is marketed as an intrinsically humble approach toward others and their cultures and creeds, but it has come to represent moral truth as essentially unknowable.

"Political correctness" is used extensively as its tool of activism. Comedian George Carlin called it "soft language" that "takes the life out of life." Masquerading as civility, PC indoctrinates people, through language and behavior, with euphemisms to obfuscate the conspicuousness of life and living in general, and it does this expressly to avoid conflict.

To claim no one can know the truth of moral knowledge is to claim there is no such thing as moral truth—a nihilistic ideal. The subject of many a philosopher, most famously the bouffant-mustachioed Friedrich Nietzsche, nihilism is the doctrine of skepticism by annihilation, most tragically of the moral, imparting itself practically as "nothing matters."

But rather than despair at the loss of meaning, the creed suggests more convincingly that there is no higher or lower significance—no hierarchy—to our earthly concerns. Well-meaning adherents will ask, "If some values are deemed 'better' than other values, how can we reach true equality?" But the question itself blithely rates our concerns the same when they are clearly not, like a discount warehouse where everything from cars to cat toys is of equal value, or, in this case, a meta–dollar store where our cares are priced to move, whether in bins of love and kindness, compassion and courage, or shelves stocked with pride and prejudice, apathy and appeasement. Prices are slashed on every belief to their cheapest—mere opinion. The indifference reveals all we need know of nihilism's philosophical essence: no one thing is of primary importance, and so anything at all can become such.

Nihilism's "no judgments" judgment can be mistaken for some sort of benevolent fairness, rather than what it rightfully is: utter confusion. As it proliferates, fidelity to truth might as well be a superpower.

The Moral as Martial: Viability

If we're going to make better decisions in the martial way, be they moral or physical, which is what prudence and vigilance are ultimately all about, we'd best not deny how better can *actually be better*.

This word *tactical* gets thrown around a lot in martial arts. Of late, I've seen "tactical combat," "tactical martial arts," even "tactical name-your-art"—it's overused and for the wrong reason, because it doesn't articulate what folks are actually trying to say.

Tactical is an adjective that describes "tactics, especially military,"[4] that are "characterized by adroit procedure" and related to "a maneuver or plan of action designed as an expedient toward gaining a desired end or temporary advantage." By this definition, everything in martial arts is already tactical: every strategy, tactic, and technique ever devised has been refined toward its aim of expedient, that is, efficient, utilization through adroit procedure. So saying your martial art is tactical is like saying you're drinking wet water. And even though buzzwords can make for better marketing, it still puts us back at our beginnings because we still have not stated what we really want to know: *how best to keep from dying.*

When we ask how to use a technique "better," we're really asking, "How ought I train to habituate protecting life?" *This* is the optimal question because it relates to the ethical prudence of decisions and judgments we make toward actual use.

So I stopped using "tactical" to mean "life protecting," since something done tactically may simply be the most efficient way to gain one's end, even at the expense of one's life. For clarity, I turned to the word *viable* to mean "in a way that protects life." *Via-* comes from the Latin *vita*, meaning "life," and describes that which is "life enabling." I now use *viable* to describe how best to protect life as we employ whatever strategy, tactic, or technique we deem necessary.

How we apply our tactical notions to make them viable is for me the dividing line that separates knowledge from wisdom, the arbitrary from the prudential. And what is far more important is the wise application of whatever knowledge one does have.

Too often, martial technique is devised, understood, or trained outside conditional use. A technique may look efficient, since it has no rough edges, but when trained against an honest partner who's trying to keep us honest, it is ineffective because we've not accounted for those conditions—we're too busy trying to do the technique "right." But too much focus on the correctness of technique is to miss the forest for the trees—the tactical aspect of martial techniques, might not keep us from dying. It's only the first act of a three-act play—the second and third acts involve identifying openings and closing them off.

Martial artists should have something much like a fashion sense, a "technical sense"—an intuition that sensibly pulls us toward techniques we have a greater chance of mastering and deters us from those that may give us more obvious trouble. This isn't to say we should only engage with the techniques or skills we find easy to use; rather, we should gravitate toward that which best represents the context of our intended use. Our manner of technique can be dictated by a variety of personal concerns: maturity, ability, athleticism, health, acumen—they all impact our mechanics and speak to how effectively and efficiently we can make those choices.

The know-how to shape techniques under real-life conditions characterizes the degree to which we understand them. This notion is akin to wearing clothes that fit us, rather than squeezing into something that doesn't, so that in practical use they do not represent a liability. Possessing a high degree of understanding involves knowing how best to embody and maximize the technical based on our individual dynamic and physical stature, rather than simply trying on various techniques. Are we fat, strong, skinny, or short? Very mobile or not so much? Being honest with ourselves in regard to strengths and vulnerabilities can indicate our direction in training, as well as calibrate us to deal with obvious realities. One of my students wears a bushel of hair on his head, an obvious target for grabs in a violent encounter, so he trains for that eventuality. This is especially important if we are working from a handicap, whether temporary or permanent.

Viability drives our overall ethic and the justness of our usage, as it speaks to how well one is able to invulnerably utilize techniques, which must include not being denied their use by the counters of an opponent.

We should seek to throw without being stabbed in the process, strike without being struck, and, of course, use weapons of any size and any shape, whether they are considered standard or have been augmented to fit our body types appropriately. All these aspects speak to ethics since we ought never unnecessarily risk ourselves or others due to poor training habits, or, worse, misinformation or misunderstanding regarding the actuality of their use.

The protector ethic is not about being reactive to the conflicts of life with preprogrammed responses. If this is the end goal of training, we're slowly programming ourselves to be overcome by countermeasures we did not or could not suspect. Repetition is important in martial training, but responses must be measured, so training is geared to understanding technique more clearly, but also to seeing, shaping, and even creating the space we need to use them in.

There is no such thing as a technique that works in and of itself. Every technique must be applied under conditions. And sharpening our perception of how best to protect life is the furthest we can reach or hope for in training them more clearly. At its core, effective training is about better decision making, so the finer our instincts regarding viability, the better the decisions we can make, and the better the survival chances we give ourselves and others.

That being said, I can think of at least five basic rules regarding viability, presented hierarchically. These are to be considered the parameters of or restrictions on how we ought to habituate ourselves physically under real-world conditions.

1. Do not be a danger to yourself.

    Be aware of threats or danger you might impose through your actions and behavior. Listen to common sense when it speaks, and heed its message.
2. Do not endanger those who need protection.

    Be a protector of others, including the enemy, if possible. Calibrate what ought to be done by context.

3. Do not allow conditions to prevent viability.

Like any good magician, know initiative to lead others by the timing of your motives.

4. Do not allow the opponent to be a danger.

Position yourself to gain the advantage of leverage and outmaneuver opponents.

5. Do not allow the opponent to prevent endangerment from your actions.

Deny your vulnerabilities and openings to those who would use them against you as you move against them.

One can't know the principles of the martial way if we only ever believe they are accomplished through the unending rules of "idealized" form, which, by the way, is exposed so obviously under the actual conditions of its use. For even if the technique is performed precisely as one has mastered it in the dojo, it's likely a square peg in a round hole if one has not first provided the safe opportunity for its use and taken advantage of that moment to the extent that the technique itself—the final piece of the puzzle—cannot be countered or stopped.

Martial techniques and their form often exist only within and are amenable to a set of controlled conditions. But to apply techniques in a manner that cannot be countered or denied under the conditions of use is to actually master their form, because *function is the form.* There is no form except that of viable functionality under real-world conditions, for how can "ideal form" be "ideal" if it cannot be actively employed under the stresses of variable conflict itself?

We can't have it both ways: either martial technique's form is a distinct and separate aspect unto itself, memorizable and useful in its exactitude and replicable for all involved, like any controlled experiment of science, or it is a malleable expression, proportional to its user and rather indistinct until it aligns to provide results under contextual conditions, like any artist might create with what they have to work with.

But there is no case in which martial form's alignment is a thing unto itself, since alignment is only possible when it references another, as in "aligned to (this thing)," which is the target of its use, and how well, where, and when it accomplishes its function by principles and internal structural resiliency under use. Even human movement is in reference not simply to itself (the body) but to the topography, environment, and, most importantly, the conditions of use—the form or alignment of walking to work in the city is completely different from climbing a mountain.

Believing in some ideal martial form is similar to thinking there is some idealized form to driving that somehow does not involve the road, its quality, the environment, weather, traffic, and any unforeseen, spontaneous, bizarre variables, such as poorly secured couches flying off the backs of pickups. In other words, the conditions that anyone can encounter at any time while performing the action known as driving. Whenever we train to drive, we are always driving, and always driving under conditions.

Defeating this rigid, idealized form for techniques means perceiving things differently. It means training in such a way that no matter what we actually do, we gain overall ability and in all areas. This means activating core principles time and again under the conditions of use to be able to apply any technique in a moment of advantage we have created for ourselves. Improving that ability has to do with setting conditions under our control, such as shaping the fighting space, much as one employs a following distance as a defensive driver.

This kind of thinking is a resurgence of old-school thought, *bushi no michi*—the path of the warrior. It is the kind of broad-minded, self-reliant warriorship that enables one to understand a plethora of tactics and strategies all aimed at undoing the enemy to protect and defend life, yet emanating from a single core or root perception, like a Rosetta stone of martial comprehension.

Growing up in a Western culture, I learned a sports-based mentality in the doing and practicing of things. "Practice makes perfect," I often heard. Later I was told that wasn't quite right—"Perfect practice makes perfect." It's well understood that if we're intent on mastering something, we must do it a lot, like, ten thousand times a lot. But there must also be a kind of perfection to this repetition, in that we must do whatever it is we are doing perfectly ten thousand times.

But here's the problem: neither of these can be relied on when it comes to training toward the protector ethic. I'd say that for many things, perhaps even most, the sports-based strategy works just fine. A professional baseball player must hit the ball tens of thousands of times to get the feel of hitting the ball well. We can wind up teaching this sports mentality because we imagine a continuum in which sports is at one end and the martial is at the other. But we should discard this notion. It isn't true.

Sports are not the opposite of martial arts any more than hunting is the opposite of war. Just imagining they are fools us into complacency. The reason why is pretty simple: the baseball player is unconcerned that, without warning, the umpire might pull a knife and stab him. He's not concerned, and rightly so, because it is not integral to the playing of baseball.

Sports exist in a measured reality—there are rules for winning. A more proper opposite to it would be something like a no-holds-barred, measured unreality, akin to video games or *Calvin and Hobbes*'s Calvinball, where indiscriminate rules are made up as you play. To this end, the better opposite of warrior arts is to take its immediate, no-second-chance reality and imagine it as the unreal—coordinated reenactment, movies, plays, and performance. "Faking it" is more properly the opposite of the martial way, and this is the great concern of mixing up our training.

Because it's intuitive, it's easy to understand how we can infuse a sports mentality into the training of martial arts. Don't get me wrong, practicing ten thousand times will get you to do that thing more dexterously than you were doing it before. But whether that thing will actually be more effective depends on how well we can apply it under real-world conditions. And the sometimes bizarre, spontaneous ever-changing reality of life is the only "condition" I am aware of that creates the complexity for being able to "play" well. In other words, the only rule is this: *change is coming.* That coming change may be good, bad, or indifferent. But the best response to that unknown is to be extemporaneously adaptive in life-preserving, viable ways.

This concept of viability is rooted in our ethical bearing, since action to protect life, whether it's our own, others', or the enemy's, is an inherently moral consideration.

Enter the Ethical Warrior

Eric Garner was a regular around a stretch of Bay Street near the Staten Island Ferry Terminal. He'd been arrested twice earlier in the year and charged for selling untaxed cigarette "loosies." The NYPD knew him well—he'd been arrested thirty times since 1980 on a variety of charges. But on July 17, 2014, he died in one final confrontation with police. Investigations followed, a grand jury, and although no one was charged for his death, the City of New York paid his family $5.9 million.

In the months after, and amid other high-profile concerns, the city began a $35 million police retraining program. But rather than assurance from officers, the public was treated to a steady drip of complaints and lousy reviews. The *New York Post* reported officers sitting (and sleeping) through eight-hour lectures, and orders to "take a deep breath" and close their eyes during tense situations. They were even made to watch clips from the Patrick Swayze movie *Road House* to teach them to "be nice."

Unfortunately, ethics can often be taught with the same sense of urgency as a forensic autopsy—cold and clinical—instead of from the impassioned plea of virtue. I don't believe anyone needs to teach police "how to ethic"; they are all perfectly capable. Cops study the law and are trained to know what is and is not just under it. And, despite what popular online memes say, most cops do join the force to serve and protect their communities.

In my opinion, much of the unethical use of force in law enforcement stems from their (too often short) stint of defensive tactics—the bushel of martial defensive and restraining techniques police officers are taught to utilize when they lay hands on suspects and criminals. The inherent problem with them was stated eloquently by Mike Tyson: "Everybody has a plan until they get punched in the face."

Blueprints are not as important as being able to form a plan and adjust it in response to context and conditions. Martial techniques are too often treated as straight answers to questions that rightfully have none—variable conflict is like that. Imagine answering the question, "What is our human purpose?" with "Grapefruit." I like grapefruit, but come on.

For cops, or anyone, to act more ethically under stress and with the confidence to lead those in conflict, they must be trained to have higher competency in their defensive tactics skills. Train officers in a physical ethic to think, speak, and act with universal values and they'll be more ethical.

Every cop ought to be a policing officer of the law and an expert in conflict mitigation and physical defense. This means training officers consistently (at least twice a week on the job) in the very kind of personal martial tactics that can allow them the physical confidence to be more ethical in their conduct and authority. Large metropolitan police agencies with thousands of officers would do well to model themselves after the Marine Corps, who figured this out—every marine is both a rifleman and a martial artist, from the recruit to the commandant.

The Marine Corps Martial Arts Program is not simply kicks and arm bars; it's infused with values that shape the combat mind-set. It's a sound strategy for generating the very kind of character and individual confidence required for leadership to make better choices. The program has promoted respect among unlike peoples, quelled violence, and stopped unnecessary killing. With the training, the marines are transforming themselves from stereotypical "killers" into "ethical warriors" with the mind-set, "No greater friend, no worse enemy."

This is quite a change after more than 240 years. Throughout all of Marine Corps history, they've been known as the dogs of war, trained to kill and set loose as necessary, from the halls of Montezuma to the shores of Tripoli. The marines perform a dirty job, battling on front lines, killing the enemy at a cost in dead and wounded comrades. Why change? Why bother? Many questioned it. Throughout all of history, humans have made war on each other. Doesn't it make sense to train a ferocious force capable of exacting a costly toll?

For more than two centuries it did. But the end of the Cold War signaled a change in strategic thinking. Pentagon soothsayers, military historians, and the forward thinkers of the armed forces could predict the future—the coming insurgencies, the asymmetrical war space, and the guerrilla lessons of Vietnam that America would relearn in blood for dozens of deployments if thinking remained unchanged. Marines were still needed, but conflicts were changing. It was the right time to ask if the marines should too.

In 1996, they did just that. They put out a call to all their heroes from the last fifty years—marines who had fought and commanded war's cruel reality by overt and covert means. The smartest, toughest, and meanest answered the call with one question in mind: How do we prepare the twenty-first-century marine?

For some, there was no debate. A good marine was a killer. Period. A rifle shooter, cannon firer, knife stabber, grenade thrower, and, most importantly, merciless foe. To make them any less would make them incapable of slogging through the blood they'll be covered with. Marines are "the few and the proud" for a reason—not all people can be marines. War's horror had demonstrated the need for malice. If touchy-feely concepts made it into marine training, it would complicate their thinking, protract their response, with inevitable results: Marines would die. Their mission would fail.

It made no matter that civilians in war zones might be left unprotected, that the strategy for victory was tallied in enemy body counts, not territory held, or lives saved. And it certainly did not matter that such "killer" training methods almost guaranteed post-traumatic stress and its disorder, the affliction that has threatened all fighting people since the Greek historian Herodotus first wrote of a soldier's self-induced blindness during the Battle of Marathon in 490 B.C.[5] The destructiveness that is PTSD is due in part to the spiritual damage humans incur for having to kill fellow human beings.

However, there were some who were not convinced the twenty-first-century marine was to be nothing but a twenty-first-century killer—Robert Humphrey. You'll recall Humphrey had seen war at its vicious and gory pinnacle as a rifle platoon commander on Iwo Jima. Humphrey proposed to the marines a brighter path than the dark road laid out by some others. He was certain the marines were ready to become the warrior-knights they were always meant to be.

Humphrey was not alone. He brought to the discussions his student of seventeen years, Jack Hoban, himself a marine. Humphrey knew early on that ethical values could only remain ethical if people were willing to stand up and physically defend them. So, in tandem with exemplary moral stories he would tell the enlisted, he reached back to his days as a Golden Gloves boxer to teach boxing on the bases he had been assigned to. Hoban has taken the philosophy many steps further. In fact, one might say he's reached back into history itself—the enigmatic and shadowy past of the Japanese ninja.

In the late 1970s, when Hoban first met Humphrey, he was already training in martial arts. But he would soon meet the second of his life's mentors. Dr. Masaaki Hatsumi of Japan was the inheritor and head of a catalog of martial lineages. But one in particular stretched back some thirty-four generations—the school of Togakure Ryu ninjutsu, art of the ninja. Hatsumi had himself been mentored by a legendary figure, Toshitsugu Takamatsu, who, like in some old movie, roamed the plains of China and Mongolia as a young man in search of adventure. He found it in death duels, in secret missions, and as a castle bodyguard for the last emperor of China.

Hatsumi had received the benefit of Takamatsu's real-world and decidedly old-school martial training and passed it on to Hoban. By 1996, Hoban was easily one of the best practitioners of it in the world. Humphrey proposed to have Hoban teach young marines the moral stories and martial arts together, providing the best chance of attaining any significant change in battlefield manner.

But Hoban was taken aback by the proposal—he remembered when he wasn't always the ethical type. Hoban was nineteen when he joined the marines. He took the Platoon Leaders Course, received a commission as a second lieutenant, then attended combat engineer school, learning to blow stuff up. By mistake, he was made acting platoon commander at the ripe age of twenty-two and wound up a series commander for drill instructors at the Marine Corps Recruit Depot in San Diego. It was 1980. Jimmy Carter was president. The Americans beat the Soviets in the "Miracle on Ice" at the Winter Olympics, the United States severed relations with Iran following the taking of American hostages, and *The Empire Strikes Back* came out.

Hoban was spending his days in a nine-to-five job on base and his nights at the Red Garter, a Cold War dive where marines, navy submariners, bikers, and foreign spies mixed in uneasy balance. "The place was unbelievable; it was like the *Star Wars* bar,"[6] Hoban said. With the naval base nearby, submariners were constantly targeted by Soviet "honey traps" collecting intelligence on submarine movements. In the years before the Berlin Wall fell, competition between Soviet and American submarines played out aggressively in the ocean depths and each night dauntlessly at the Garter. Smack in the middle of intrigue, biker fights, spilled hooch, and loose women, a gruff Hoban felt right at home.

That is, once he had "mentally killed" everyone in the room.

Hoban could never relax until he had sized up the place and every-one in it. He observed whatever locals might be there and assessed their threat to him, then mentally formulated a defense. He'd envisage tossing some navy "squid" into the wall, breaking a biker's arm, or smashing a bottle over another's head. Once he felt he'd addressed every threat, he could sit down and enjoy his beer.

Hoban had the Vietnam-era GI Bill and decided to go back to school for an MBA. A required course was Cross-cultural Conflict Resolution in Business, and the professor was a tweed-jacketed, elbow-patch-wearing, typical seventies touchy-feely guy: Humphrey.

When he first met him, Hoban could barely keep his eyes from roll-ing. The four-hour course met twice weekly, and Humphrey used every minute of the first class to interview each student. When he finally reached Hoban, the older man took one look at his high-and-tight haircut and said, "So, you're a marine, I guess?"

"What gave it away, Pops?" thought Hoban.

"I was a marine too. A rifle platoon commander on Iwo Jima."

He might as well have said he had walked on the moon. Hoban, like the hairs on his neck, sat up a little straighter.

Hoban took a liking to Humphrey and his commonsense ways. But Hoban was a tough nut, maybe too tough. "When I knew [Hum-phrey] in San Diego, he was starting to get irritated by me, I could tell. I was such a macho hard ass, you have no idea. Marines, training in martial arts, I think I'm a ninja, and I've done all kinds of . . . non-sense. Stuff I don't want printed. What it had turned me into was a very hard, harsh person." So Humphrey asked a favor of Hoban. The next time he caroused at the Red Garter, instead of arriving and men-tally murdering the room, think this instead: *everyone is safer because I'm here.*

Hoban eventually returned to the Red Garter. He walked into the din and intrigue, the threats and dangers, looked over the room and said to himself: everyone is safer because I'm here. Nobody cared, of course, and the drinking and carousing didn't stop. But Hoban felt different—better than he had in a long time. It was an epiphany. And it changed him.

Humphrey's understanding of the human condition was so vast, he impressed even Hatsumi, who bestowed on him an honorary tenth-degree black belt, the highest level of mastery. In fact, on the wall of Hatsumi's dojo in Japan is a photo of Humphrey and his "Warrior Creed":

Wherever I walk, everyone is safer.
Wherever I am, anyone in need has a friend.
Whenever I return home, everyone is happy I am there.
It's a better life!

Hoban is now president of Resolution Group International, a company that teaches ethics and conflict resolution to law enforcement and the military. These days, Hoban is very much the big-brother type: popular, wise with council, but edgy too. He suffers no fools because he can't—he's out to save lives.

Law enforcement is doing its own soul searching, and it's no mystery why—poor decisions and actions in law enforcing make headlines that the media are all too happy to exploit, even though it overshadows the good work done by law enforcement's majority.

Cops require a method to form viable, tactical habits and must be trained in it consistently in order to achieve its intrinsic benefits. But those sound habits must come from deference to universal values, which, when recognized, always achieve the one thing everyone—cops, civilians, and criminals—can appreciate: respect for the value of their lives.

This has to do with how they use their bearing, attitude, and confidence, including body language, for they directly impact whether situations worsen or de-escalate. A firm knowledge of human nature always provides an edge to those who would deal with its turbulence. The reempowering of police should vitalize their personal behavior to serve and protect themselves, as well as the rest of us.

Hoban's message resonates. He knows martial training to physically protect self and others is the best way to instill and calibrate ethical values, especially the Marine Corps's core values: honor, courage, and commitment. But he says, "That's when the trouble started."

Don't terrorists talk honor? Ever heard of an "honor killing" or "honor among thieves"? Is that the same kind of honor as the one the Marine Corps values? What about courage? Don't terrorists believe it's courageous to sacrifice themselves by blowing up and killing innocents? And they talk commitment to their beliefs. Are these values morally equivalent? And if not, why not? What separates the values, morals, and ethics of US Marines from those of terrorists who target innocent people? So the Marine Corps had to ask: *Do they share the same values as terrorists?*

Marines knew their values were different. If a terrorist shoots a marine and closes, that terrorist will kill that marine. But when a marine shoots a terrorist, if the terrorist is no longer a threat, the marine will render first aid. And if the marine kills that unarmed terrorist, the marine could face arrest and be charged with murder. Does anyone think terrorists are putting their people on trial for killing in cold blood?

There is no moral equivalency. The values of the marines are different, but they needed to articulate why in a basic, easily understandable way. Hoban's mentor, Humphrey, had his own theory. The "Dual-Life Value" recognizes the balance and imbalance between self and others. It holds that we consciously or subconsciously value our life (self) and the lives of loved ones (others) and can reason to value strangers by extension, even those outside our group whose behavior we disagree with. Humphrey said it best: "Obviously, it does not mean that people are not different in almost all measurable ways. You may be bigger than I am, smarter than I, better built, stronger, faster in mind and body, better looking, possess a more popular skin color, etc. Nonetheless, in one way, in a way that eclipses all others in controlling importance, I AM YOUR EQUAL: MY LIFE AND THE LIVES OF MY LOVED ONES ARE AS IMPORTANT TO ME AS YOURS ARE TO YOU."[7]

Do different people have different morals? Of course. Morals are based on values, and one person's values are different from another's. In America, we value freedom, liberty, democracy, and the pursuit of happiness. Do terrorists cherish those values? Not likely, values are relative. In parts of the world, women are considered unequal and brutally subjugated by men because that's their cultural value. Does that make it okay? Moral relativism says we can't know for sure, and, rather than challenge our thinking to discover truth, plenty of folks are willing to do what's practical—read, easy—and just "go along to get along." Being practical is great when you build a deck, but it's not so great when you're making moral decisions because it merely sidesteps the big questions. And big questions are big for a reason: they take up so much space that they're awfully hard to ignore.

If we're going to train in the martial way, we need to know right from wrong—we may have to harm or kill to protect ourselves or someone else. If we fail to act, or overreact and take life when we don't need to, it will haunt us the rest of our days. Our military and law enforcement are taught how to fight, but they are sometimes woefully unprepared for the spiritual damage that occurs in conflict—the damage we do to ourselves for having to fight and kill fellow human beings.

Throughout history, the warrior has been charged with the delivery and security of "better" and "safer." But how can we manage this if we are ignorant, relativistic, or dishonest regarding the truth of better and safer? We have to know the difference. For the protector ethic, warriorship is the means to know.

At its heart, martial training is a search for moral values. But training alone will not make us moral, any more than simply going to church makes us good. Ethics are morals in action, but they don't count if we keep them to ourselves. And without ethics, martial arts are just a bunch of yelling, jumping, and swinging stuff around—a selfish endeavor, if not for the responsibility they bestow.

Vigilance

I can't remember the first time I saw this, perhaps as a lad thumbing through George Kirby's numerous volumes of *Jujitsu*, but I didn't appreciate it much at the time. I came across it again recently, only this time it was called the "golden rule of combat" and was supposedly from an old book by Jigoro Kano, the founder of judo.

> Your most powerful weapon, applied to your opponent's greatest weakness, at his time of maximum vulnerability.

A helpful paraphrase of it: "Our best shot at his weakest point when he's least ready." I tell ya, it all sounds great. Most powerful weapon, weakness, maximum vulnerability—all the right and good stuff. But I'm gonna disagree with it, not because I think it's wrong, or even because I don't think it's right enough—surely there are folks who will testify to its truth.

I don't care for it because it perceives things exactly backward, like looking into a mirror looking at the world—we experience it as an image of reality instead of reality itself. If we aren't clear about what is actual, then we can't be clear about how to deal with it.

Training goals become misguided when what we value most ought not be most valued. When this happens, we wind up with a defensive strategy that doesn't hold up under stress. If we're placing technique at the top of our list, whether that's memorization or the "most powerful weapon," we wind up confused. Like a pyramid on its head, it's not that we can't find its point of balance, there is one, of course, it's that it is too easy to tip over.

First off, I'm not certain what my most powerful weapon is. I think in terms of opportunities I can take advantage of, and insert whatever I have available at the time. That may be a right cross, front kick, or an improvised weapon, but I'll only know that at the time of use and the conditions I'm under. What's clearly more valuable than a personal WMD is creating a moment of my choosing I can exploit to weaken or destroy an opponent's ability to out-position and gain leverage on me, rather than merely waiting for the chance to throw my "hammer."

I also don't know what my opponent's greatest weakness is, whether that's instable shoulders, bad knees, or a heart condition. An opportunistic weakness is just that—opportune. And let's be honest, using my most powerful weapon against their greatest weakness may not actually do a thing, since "most powerful" is abstract and may not actually be powerful at all, just powerful for me.

But here's the most telling part: at his time of maximum vulnerability (read: imbalance). *His time?* Sounds like I'm waiting for his balance to imbalance itself. Listen, by the time we recognize imbalance, it's too late—it'll be corrected before we ever get a chance to exploit it. So why isn't this notion on *my time* instead of his time? Let's not understate clarity. This notion ought to be in reference to me, since I'm the one to dictate it to the opponent. That's the only way it's big enough to see and long enough to take advantage of because I know where and when it will occur.

Writing my own "golden rule," I'd start and end with *time*, as in "timing," as in the "interval." The interval is the discontinuity between what the opponent has actually done—his action—and what he wants to do—his intention and the requisite tactical maneuvers taken in that moment. Remember, fights don't start with a first strike—fights start from the position to strike first. It's like in war—when armies battle, they don't shoot first; they maneuver to position themselves to shoot. If we're using an OODA (observe, orient, decide, act) loop to map this out, the interval would be between "act" (the last part) and "observe" (the first part)—conflict consists not of just one OODA loop but a cascading series of them.

At the very least, let's flip the saying:

When he's least ready, strike his weakest point with your best shot.

This already sounds better to me. It's cleaner because it follows how we actually need to operate and clearer simply because we oriented first for time, the moment of action. The interval needs to be first, since in reality it always comes first. "Timing is everything" because time is the space for action to occur.

Now, let's refine:

> When he's made least ready, target any weak point with capable technique.

Now we're active instead of passive, making him less ready instead of waiting for him to be such. We make him less ready by our maneuvering in the interval.

A little better:

> When he is made to move against an opportunity we have created, exploit a weakness in his position with techniques that cannot be countered or stopped.

Okay, now we're in deep, making him least ready by giving him a golden opportunity he simply can't pass up and targeting the weaknesses inherent in his actions in moving against us. If we take advantage of a weak point and ride it, whatever technical means we are using become increasingly difficult to counter or stop, provided we know how to apply them that way.

Better still:

> Lead the opponent by his motives to take advantage of a created vulnerability, shape his resulting action in the interval between what he wanted and what he has instead been made to do, and take advantage of his ensuing action with applied techniques that cannot be denied their use.

Expose his motives by your vulnerability—an opportunity for us, since now we can be sure of what he will do—and take advantage of the physical contradiction he's left with. What he originally wanted is not what he has been made to do because we're still maneuvering, but now he's following us. The context of our conditions—whether we are escaping or subduing this person—is key, as it dictates response, and continued maneuvering gives us advantage, providing we have the training to shape the moment to that end. Our technique is then simply a matter of judging the changing conditions to achieve the outcome we need or want.

Best:

Initiate his motives by self-risking, create a physical contradiction between what he wanted and what he has been made to do by repositioning, and when he attempts recovery, exploit that weakness with just enough leverage to undo his original motive completely and achieve our contextual outcome.

By initiating our ethic, the timing of our motivating values, we also initiate the opponent's action by his motive. In short, we lead by giving others the example we want them to be led by. Conflict resolution is a matter of displaying leadership under stress, whether that's with your team at work or against stacked odds in a violent street encounter. Creating opportunities that opponents can be lured by is the surest means to defeat them—humans have only been doing this in hunting and fighting since the dawn of time.

Trapping people inside their own mistakes often forces them to extricate themselves from those mistakes before returning to the fight—a costly move. The action alone is enough to cause an opening to appear so they can be undone and we can achieve our desired outcome by context, whether that's escaping, interceding on another's behalf, or subduing for control or arrest.

Our mind-set plays an incredibly vital role in the formation of this kind of self-awareness. If we are simply trying to master a set of physical skills that have been gathered together to form a martial art, it holds no potential except in whatever physical strength we infuse it with. How much faster or more powerfully can we actually punch or kick or joint lock or throw as we grow older? And certainly our understanding of technique will not protect us—it might in fact give us a false sense of confidence.

But if we embrace this sort of prudential vigilance, we can learn to live and think and look at the world from a mindful concern that is both tactical and viable. In fact, we might, in a sense, see the world the same as early humans viewed theirs, where you lived cautiously each and every day to protect yourself and others.

Making better physical decisions and coming to clearer judgments to prudentially assess our martial choices is a practiced commitment of clarifying and protecting the good. And it is through that commitment that we can reach the kind of vigilance that is needed for the protector ethic.

NOTES

1. "Truth," The Free Dictionary, accessed October 23, 2017, http://www.thefreedictionary.com/truth.
2. "Spit-take," Wikipedia, August 21, 2016, accessed October 23, 2017, https://en.wikipedia.org/wiki/Spit-take#cite_note-0.
3. Later, I wrote this to the student who spoke up: "A few weeks ago, when [our Professor] made the awkward (I'm being kind) comparison between choosing to save a human life from fire and choosing to save a 'priceless' painting, you spoke up rather forcefully, saying, in essence, human life is 'out of bounds' when considering these kinds of decisions. On some level you knew the comparison itself was wrong. But why? Was it because you knew the guard's 'nexus of cares'? His want to become manager? His great regard for his stamp collection? His love for his children or grandchildren? Of course not. You knew none of this, and none of it was necessary for you to know the comparison was immoral. However, you did know one thing: the guard is alive and in so being values his life just as you value yours. And if we don't want others equating our life with their relative cares or values, then clearly it is not allowable for us to do so to them. The guard is a person, has agency, has autonomy, and is self-determined because he is alive. And, therefore, so are we."
4. "Tactical," Dictionary.com, accessed October 23, 2017, http://www.dictionary.com/browse/tactical.

5. "Epizelus, the son of Cuphagoras, an Athenian, was in the thick of the fray, and behaving himself as a brave man should, when suddenly he was stricken with blindness, without blow of sword or dart; and this blindness continued thenceforth during the whole of his after life. The following is the account which he himself, as I have heard, gave of the matter: he said that a gigantic warrior, with a huge beard, which shaded all his shield, stood over against him; but the ghostly semblance passed him by, and slew the man at his side. Such, as I understand, was the tale which Epizelus told." Herodotus, *The Persian Wars*, Book 6, Erato, 6.11.

6. James V. Morganelli, "Ethical Warrior," *Black Belt*, June 2011, 54–58.

7. Robert L. Humphrey, *Values for a New Millennium* (Maynardville, TN: Life Values, 2005), 50 (emphasis in the original).

4

To Act: Courage as Rectitude

The Storms of Human Nature

"I got one hundred feet, everything was an orange hue, there was snow in my face, I couldn't see anything, I turned around and couldn't see the bus and I thought I was going to die."[1]

Lindsey Wilson wasn't kidding. She was trapped by the storm of the century—a blizzard seen once every fifty years—thundering across half the nation, from New Mexico to Boston into eastern Canada. It killed twenty-four people and caused damage in excess of $1 billion.

On January 31, 2011, the Groundhog Day storm—"Snowmageddon" in the Midwest—dumped twenty inches on Chicago by four thirty in the afternoon, causing whiteout. Twenty-four-year-old Wilson was aboard a rush-hour bus now stranded on the city's iconic Lake Shore Drive after drifting snow caused a jackknife that corked up the thoroughfare.

Once movement ceased, seventy-mile-per-hour winds whipped drifts as high as the bus and buried 1,500 other vehicles. Some of these folks were less than a mile from home and would spend the night inside their cars. Wilson and a few others left the bus at one point to seek shelter in nearby buildings, only to march right back when they lost their bearings. She spent the next twelve hours with a handful of strangers waiting for rescue by snowmobile firefighters.

As a Chicagoan, I remember the snow, shoveling it mostly, and the eerie calm the morning after, when the streets were impassable and only a few shuffling souls were out seeking basic goods. Lake Shore Drive looked like an aircraft boneyard as wind blew ice and apathy into abandoned cars, burying them like toys in a sandy beach. Folks waited hours for rescue, their gasoline long extinguished and their heaters now just open vents to the punishment outside.

Did they have blankets with them? A little food? A heat source, like a candle? And matches to light it? What about a pair of extra gloves, or socks, let alone an extra sweater or jacket? Had it not been for first responders, Chicago's leadership, the brain-dead trust who refused to shut down Lake Shore Drive even when they knew it would become impassable before they could clear it, would have been the end of them.

When we think of survival, most folks—who are not dummies by any means—tend to think of being lost in a national forest or their Camry's transmission stutter to a smoky end in Death Valley. But less than a mile from home? No, most folks typically don't worry about surviving their daily commute.

As any Midwesterner will affirm, it is not strange or pointless to actively prepare for acts of nature. We, as its inhabitants, are subject to its will. And we cannot negotiate or bribe it into snowing, or raining, or tornadoing some other time. Storms happen. We know they are inevitable, and we know we must deal with them in sober, smart ways, which grants us the best chance to withstand their arrival and duration. No one living in Blizzardville, Flood Grove, or Tornado Alley thinks it unwise, let alone a waste of time, to prepare for such.

Storms also happen in human nature. And just as we would be remiss in dismissing Mother Nature's inevitable arrival, we do ourselves and others—some of whom we might care a great deal about—a disservice when we do not plan, soberly or smartly, to deal with the inevitable storms of the often fragile and volatile human condition. There are consequences for abstention.

Who would dispute that if we wandered into a snowstorm without a coat or grabbed a red-hot coal with bare hands, we would risk becoming sick from cold or burned by fire? Each of us learns early in life that disrespecting nature bears costs. Disrespect the weather, or fire, or any number of natural phenomenon, and one will suffer—not might, will—consequences for disrespect. Results can vary from physical harm, in which the body is injured or destroyed, to mental, as in phobic response to certain stimuli. Disorienting ourselves from the actuality of the nature we live in, as well as the human nature we live by, risks life, limb, and limbic health.

The storms of human nature speak to the essence of what this work is about: to embody the protector ethic by rediscovering the self-evident. If we are going to do more than theorize martial ethics, and physically embrace them by all means, then we must come to terms with a certainty: truth, in all its weight and consequence, is only identified in the world *as it actually is*, not the world we want or wish there to be.

The martial way demands clarity, and it must be driven by this standard of truth. If it is not, we risk ourselves and others by training, physically and perceptually, to become a liability; one that not only misperceives ethical choices and mistrains physical principles, but can even become physically immobilized by the confounding effect of violence.

It is courage that grants dependability for rectitude, the steadfastness of our behavior and warriorship, and the final virtue for the protector ethic. And for the warrior, there is no greater virtue than courage as rectitude, since it is the key to manifest action to do, that which calms our nerves to withstand the inexplicable acts of human storms, and steadies our legs for battle in the stand against its evil.

Evil

In the early hours of Sunday, June 12, 2016, just before closing, three hundred people packed the Orlando, Florida, nightclub Pulse and were readying to leave. They took final sips of drinks and said good night to friends. Saturday was Latin Night at the normally gay club, and the previous evening had seen locals flock in to dance bachata.

At 2:00 a.m., gunshots cracked the din of DJ music, there were screams, and twenty-nine-year-old Omar Mateen, a young American born to an Afghan family, entered with a set of firearms and opened up on the crowd. At 2:09 a.m., the club posted a single message online, "Everyone get out of pulse and keep running." Over the next three hours, Mateen shot more than one hundred people, killing forty-nine of them. In calls lasting a near total of thirty minutes to 911 operators and negotiators, he claimed allegiance to terrorist groups, even posting shout-outs online during the attack such as, "Taste the Islamic state vengeance." Amid the innocent clubgoers who lay wounded and dying, he lamented US bombings of Syria and Iraq and claimed the same to reporters at a local news station when he called them.

The following Tuesday, the Graves family, from Elkhorn, Nebraska, were enjoying their vacation at a Disney resort, also in Orlando. Their youngest, Lane, just two years old, was wading in foot-deep water in the Seven Seas Lagoon when he was literally ripped from the grip of his father by an alligator.

The twin horrors gripped America. The nation staggered.

Folks were shocked by an alligator attacking a child, especially at a fancy resort for families and fun. In the aftermath, "How did this happen?" was a demand, and Disney was made to answer it. But no fair-minded person asked the other big question—why?

"Why did this happen?" seeks motive. It was not asked because everyone, on some level, already knew the answer: alligators are alligators. Nature's prime directive is survival. This single-mindedness is often considered cruel by human standards, but it's a given. Thus, the answer to any motive of nature is usually itself: Why alligator? Because alligator.

We know the reasons animals act like the animals they are, be it their environment or sociobiology. But their motives? Undomesticated animal motives are driven by the life force of their existence. They are, by definition, devoid of self-reflection and unrepentant. We may not like what we see and experience of the natural world, but because it bears the seal of nature, we can square its manner with the "circle of life" and even endure its destruction, be it storms or animal attacks.

Not so with Omar Mateen. His attack not only broke the American heart, but dealt a blow to some so severe as to cause a psychic U-turn, an inversion eliciting self-loathing despair that cries out to know whatever it was *we did* to deserve such a fate. This is the result of comprehending horror, and trying to reconcile its capricious and arbitrary motives with the carnage in its wake. Doing so can entrap the human mind and even send us into a spiral of confusion and inaction. Under the immeasurable stress of deadly violence, like a mass shooting, this could cause us to physically shut down in the very moment we need to keep moving.

The nightclub and alligator attacks were each in their own way perfect examples of the existential threat that both philosophers and theologians have agonized over for millennia—the problem of evil. Evil as a concept is such for at least two reasons: first, its perceived destructive impact on human life, and, second, its inevitable consequence, suffering. The extraordinary difference between the events that week in June highlighted a fundamental distinction: one was moral evil, done by man, and the other was nonmoral or so-called natural evil, due to nature.

Rectitude comes from regular physical training against the intimate danger of violence that has perpetually savaged mankind. The first lesson in this training, and its most demanding, is admission of a grim, twofold reality: one, evil, by way of human and natural endeavor and in all its variety and repulsion, is an exigent force in this world, as much as any expression of hope or love. And two, it is irresolvable and unavoidable in its advent.

Unfortunately, many folks are so fearful of this basic truth, they will lie and deceive so as not to deal with its implications. This is self-destruction as ravenous as the Ouroboros that eats itself by the tail. But in the end, there is no avoiding the simple truth of the matter: a man murdered for his own specific reasons, and, like any animal of nature, he was single-mindedly cruel, devoid of self-reflection, and unrepentant.

If the answer to the motives of nature is always itself, then this must also be the case for human nature: just as there is no fixing alligators of their alligatoring, there is no fixing human evil.

The "Good" of Evil

Now, perhaps you choose not to subscribe intellectually to evil as a concept. Or you feel that labeling what are arguably sociopathic actions and tragic incidents with such a theologically loaded term as *evil* distracts from some pragmatic clarity of what to actually do about them. You would not be alone.

Within organized philosophy there exists something called *evil-skepticism*, the adherents of which feel that use of the term proliferates supernatural influence. They also point to its vague definitions, often tied to dark and spooky metaphysics, which too often allow it to be drafted as a trigger for legal and political concerns, such as when President Ronald Reagan called the Soviet Union an "evil empire."

Friedrich Nietzsche felt the term *evil* should be abandoned, as it entreated the weak only to hold back the strong. He famously said, "The great epochs of our life come when we gain the courage to rechristen our evil as what is best in us."[2] Harvard psychology professor Steven Pinker wrote of the "myth of pure evil."[3] "The reason that this is a myth (when seen through psychological spectacles)," he says, "is that evil in fact is perpetrated by people who are mostly ordinary, and who respond to their circumstances, including provocations by the victim, in ways they feel are reasonable and just."[4] Pinker's conception can be traced to the phrase "banality of evil," originally coined by Hannah Arendt during the 1963 trial of Adolf Eichmann, who you'll recall was the chief architect of the Nazi Holocaust. The phrase is meant to convey the mundane, everydayness with which some commit unspeakably evil acts (perhaps because they've "rechristened" them). It captures Eichmann's unremarkableness and his thoughtless lack of introspection regarding his workaday decisions to condemn millions to torturous labor and the ovens of death camps.

The truth of conflict is akin to a force of nature—cold and indifferent to our concerns. We either make a conscious choice to prepare ourselves for its impending arrival or suffer the agonies of "too little, too late." It is exactly the kind of conflict good folks never wish to think about, let alone discuss—the threatening and potentially violent kind.

Regardless of how we feel about evil as a concept, it is precisely the established difference between an act of the natural world and the malicious actions of a member of our own species—nature versus nurture, if you will—that allowed only one of the events that fateful June to be readily reconciled—Lane's death. The reason was a simple one: there was no fear of truth in that case—it was as plain as simple addition. An act of nature. But fear of truth in Mateen's case was actually something much more primal: fear of conflict.

The martial way cannot authentically exist without recognition of the truth of moral evil and acceptance of its unforgiving certainty. Moral evil contains an inherent reality that natural evil does not— conflict between humans. Aggressive human conflict stokes our fears and vulnerabilities, assaults our sense of personal rights, liberty, and dignity in a way that no torrential storm, disease, or act of nature can achieve. Rape, robbery, and murder speak not only to the failures of the human condition but also of a ghastly emotion, uncontained in any storm—malevolence. No one ever need feel targeted by a tornado, but human-on-human violence traumatizes.

121

Lieutenant Colonel Dave Grossman calls human conflict the "universal human phobia" in his book *On Combat*: "When violence does happen to us, it devastates us. It shatters us. . . . We do not expect that one of the millions of Americans we interact with in an average lifetime will try to kill us. We simply cannot lead our lives expecting that every human we meet might try to kill us. So when someone does try to kill us, it is simply not right and, if we are not careful, it can destroy us."[5] Trauma can last for years, triggering survival emotions such as anxiety, fear, and depression arising from guilt and humiliation. It often results in post-traumatic stress.

Notwithstanding myths about its purity, or the vagueness of its character, moral evil is the recurrent bold footnote in the book of man. Far from being a useless or counterproductive term, and in spite of the benevolence that we aspire and are inspired to, moral evil is our shared destructive impulse and base instinct to do one thing more egregiously than anything else: dehumanize, whether others or the self. The moral repugnancy of the Holocaust and genocide in any time defies our best efforts to describe or understand it as "bad" or "very bad." I suppose Reagan could have called the Soviet Union the "really, really awful empire," but "evil" summed up the interminable bloody stain of the despotic torment and slaughter of a hundred million people during communism's twentieth-century reign of terror.

If there is "good" to be found in the concept of evil, then it is that its malevolence and destructive outcomes stand in direct proportion to the depth with which we imbue life with sacred dignity. As the sharpest proof of the devastating forces at the root of human suffering, the term *evil* is indispensable as a means of validation because it is, at its least, antithetical to our sustainment and protection.

Evil defined by any standard, be it supernatural, theological, secular, mythological, or that of Screwtape himself, is still characterized by negation. Like cold is to heat, or darkness to light, evil's true measure is not its absence of "goodness" or "benevolence" but its absence of respect for the sacrosanct value of human life. This connectivity to our common humanity is viscerally felt by the sense of injustice, even personal guilt, experienced when life is stripped uncompromisingly from the innocent and the heroic alike.

Evil not only acknowledges the intensity of that violation but also gives voice to the historical and anthropological DNA of free will, woven into our human nature. The so-called banality of evil underscores the point, since part of what it means to be human is that everyone and anyone is capable of evil's wicked methods. And even if not express candidates for its ways, some may surely use ignorance or outright lies to shun, cover up, and otherwise disavow its conduct and costs, if only to avoid contact with it, as well as keep hidden from the burden of obligation to stand against it.

In the conclusion of his book *The Myth of Evil*, Phillip Cole states, "'Evil' is a black-hole concept which gives the illusion of explanation, when what it actually represents is the failure to understand."[6] Even as he argues for the term's abandonment, Cole nails evil's description as inexplicable. It is. Evil's motives are contrarational and cannot be entirely reconciled, just like any act of nature, only accepted for what they are. As John Kekes writes, "Psychologizing with the object of explaining evil is in a different class because it is an active force preventing our sensibility from facing evil."[7]

This is exactly the problem with trying to understand and make sense of evil acts—they defy our best intentions of trying to rationalize the irrational. Examination and inquiry require some form of tolerance in any prolonged study of its depravity. And over time, this can blunt our sensibilities, numbing us to atrocity. Just ask the good folks of the City of Chicago, who have yet to deal effectively with an intolerable murder rate that far outpaces military deaths in US theaters of war. People numb themselves to conflict to protect their psyches.

As we strive for steadfastness through fortitude and courage, we are confronted by the reality of evil's customs and are dared to comprehend their lesson: evil's truth is conflict itself. And conflict is so frightening to most that it bars them from holding values and beliefs or

123

taking positions that offer any challenge to it. When we cannot escape it, we'll often delude ourselves and even lie to others to convince them of its absence.

For protectors, taking the world as it is must be the first step to resolving that confusion.

From Sun Tzu to Sensei Obvious

As much as we believe we do, we too often do not take the world as it is—we can't help it; we're human. We project on its situations and people our own values and ways of knowing. We do this as a means of orienting ourselves in a world that is sometimes in conflict with our values, and we can't help but succumb to a normalcy bias, the belief that we are somehow protected from calamity and violence and, in a wider sense, from the unknown itself.

But in taking the world as it is, we accept every brutal reality, and all the variables and changes, both overt and hidden, that the human condition can possibly concoct to aim harm at its fellow man. Change and its variables are the singular law of the open world. To discard this notion, or make oneself numb to its particularities, would be to train oneself to see the world *not* as it is but as one wishes it were or wants it to be.

A few years back, Sam Harris, who has a PhD in neuroscience, wrote a piece called "The Truth about Violence," outlining his principles of self-defense.[8] Though well meaning, it was a master class in confirmation and normalcy bias, perpetuating the myth that folks will naturally respond to and meet physical conflict and violence. His three principles are the following:

1. Avoid dangerous people and dangerous places.
2. Do not defend your property.
3. Respond immediately and escape.

Upon first reading these points may seem reasonable. Harris states, "The primary goal of self-defense is to avoid becoming the victim of violence. The best way to do this is to not be where violence is likely to occur."

Now, I hope it doesn't take a PhD in neuroscience to realize we should "avoid dangerous people and places." Harris's first admonition reminds me of answers coaches give to sportscaster questions about their game-day strategy: "I think if we score more points than the other team, we'll win." That's some Sun Tzu right there.

It would be great if, by controlling our location and behavior, everyone could simply avoid the people and places of violence. If we could, we wouldn't even need to consider our personal defense. But the fact is that conflict and violence can occur anywhere at all, from the biggest cities to the smallest towns, where we work, live, drive, shop, eat, sleep, and travel—no matter how we're behaving. We can never be certain where or how conflict and violence will occur. And if we could, we would avoid it without question.

The word *principle* means, "a comprehensive and fundamental law." Even if we take Harris's first maxim to mean, "Don't behave in a way that invites violence," he never explains or advises how to alter the way we were behaving before. There's no principle here; it's just good advice. But say we take this first notion at face value. What if we reside in a dangerous place, like folks in Chicago neighborhoods trapped by spiraling violence? What's the plan, then? We should not go home or go out? We should move? What if we can't?

Many people believe, inaccurately, they are out of range of conflict and violence. That their security, location, or means create a green zone around them and those they care about. But this is as silly a notion as believing one is out of range of the weather. Buying into this, even tacitly, is the rational equivalent of sticking one's head in the sand. Eventually, the tide comes in.

It is facetious to think there could be particular rules of assent or belief that, if simply complied with, could relieve us of the burden of human conflict. Anything claiming this mantle only ever avails itself of the most obvious command, like Monty Python's instructions for how to play the piano: move your fingers about, making sure they hit the right notes in the correct order—like a pianist does. The British comedians would have mightily approved of Harris's advice. Picture a skit called "Monty Python's Rules of Self-defense." First rule: avoid dangerous people and dangerous places. Second rule: maintain strict adherence to first.

Harris's next point is "Do not defend your property." Right. I get where he's going with this—your wallet isn't worth your life. Got it. But could there ever be a case in which we're justified in defending property? What if that property is life protecting or life sustaining? The real question is, is there any property worth dying for? Say you're carrying a cure for cancer in your backpack and you're mugged. The loss of this prototype cure means the deaths of thousands, maybe more. Maybe people you love. Would that be worth fighting or dying for? Harris uses the example of not defending your vehicle from vandals— just call the police he says. Sounds reasonable. That is, unless you need your car to evacuate your family from a looming hurricane.

We don't need to make up hypotheticals. Folks trapped in their homes in the aftermath of Hurricane Katrina in Louisiana waited upward of a week before they saw their first police officer, and in the meantime they had to contend with roving bands of armed looters looking to steal food, water, and guns. It happened in Haiti too after the earthquake of 2010. Take the 2011 riots in London or America— some shop owners turned out to defend their small businesses from fiery ruin. If your business is how you feed your family, and without it they may go hungry and become destitute, guess what? You show up with a baseball bat. Or a shotgun. And some did. Sales of baseball bats in England on Amazon.com rose 5,000 percent during the riots. My point is there are cases that could be made for defending property. So, again, this is not some immutable principle of self-defense.

Harris's last point is "Respond immediately and escape," and he backs it up with lines like, "You have no alternative but to explode into action, whatever the risk." And, "Strike preemptively without telegraphing your moves." Listen, I am a lifelong martial artist who's trained for forty years on my moves and I have trouble doing all of this.

I'm all for avoidance and escaping, and Harris is not wrong here. The gut response of anyone whose life is threatened by another person is to escape. This is natural. Everyone tries to get away. It's when folks can't get away that things get complicated. We've heard of "fight or flight." Well, when "flight" is not an option, "fight" is not necessarily first on everyone's to-do list. Even if attacking our attacker is an option, the majority of people will not do it. The mistake Harris and many of those who read his piece—and who will likely never consistently train—are making is they are taking it for granted that they'll fight back and confirming a bias they do not know to be false.

Fighting back seems reasonable, and is easy to assume. But it spits in the face of reality when rough, violent people are commanding we do something we would never voluntarily do. When safety and life are threatened by other humans and escape is not possible, some folks posture, or put up a good front, trying to talk their way out. But most people will submit and just give in and give up. *If there's a "truth about violence," this is it.*

Survivors of school and mass shootings who "played dead" later recalled in interviews that they just gave up and "waited to die." They couldn't flee, they didn't counterattack, they didn't posture; they submitted. Submission is the baseline response, the predictable human behavior of most people when faced with life-threatening danger from another human. They don't want to get hurt, they don't want to die, and, if they cannot escape, they will give up rather than fight. Bear in mind, I'm not talking about receiving defensive wounds—everyone protects themselves instinctively—but rather about engaging an aggressor for the purposes of escape or any other end.

This response is what the majority of regular people can be expected to do, and it is not limited to the untrained masses. Jeff Cooper, the quintessential man's man, a marine in World War II and Korea who was responsible for what is known as the modern technique of defensive shooting, wrote, "Any man who is a man may not, in honor, submit to threats of violence. But many men who are not cowards are simply unprepared for the fact of human savagery. They have not thought about it . . . and they just don't know what to do. When they look right into the face of depravity or violence they are astonished and confounded."[9]

If we wish to counteract this "confounding" response to the storms of human nature, the majority of humanity that is not born with a Chuck Norris beard and fists named "law" and "order" must study, prepare, and train to learn a new and different behavior. No one can simply put a checkmark in the box next to "elbow to the solar plexus, kick to the groin." Hell, even Cooper and Norris got themselves trained. But to expect that the average person is capable of doing so and will do so with no training is not simply misguided; it's dangerous because it perpetuates this myth of fighting back.

And this myth is not isolated to those under direct threat. David Brooks's November 14, 2011, *New York Times* piece "Let's All Feel Superior" mentions Normalcy Bias, Motivated Blindness, and Bystander Effect as explanations for why a Penn State graduate student didn't physically stop Coach Jerry Sandusky when he walked in on him raping a ten-year-old in the shower. The fact is that even good folks who witness violence, in a crowd or individually, have an extraordinary apprehension about helping those on the receiving end. They won't call 911 or provide aid, and they certainly will not lay hands on the perpetrators.

If you'd like a preview of your own gut reaction, you should do yourself a favor: jump on the net, look up "streetfight," and watch a dozen videos of actual, brutal confrontations. These are just the kinds of people we are concerned about defending ourselves from. Now, place yourself in the opposite position—would you help any of these people? Call police? Stop a victim's bleeding? Jump into the fray? If not, you're "normal." But if you're someone who usually goes to the aid of others, then chances are you will come to your own aid. In fact, aiding others is great training to help ourselves.

I'm not saying this baseline behavior is moral or ethical. I am saying it should be expected. And if we wish to change our expected behavior, our "normal" response, then we have but one choice: train ourselves to behave differently. When high schoolers tackled Kip Kinkle at Thurston High during a murderous shooting spree on May 21, 1998, they may or may not have had previous martial training. But they all played football—a heavy, physical contact sport—and in that, they were all "trained."

Conflict-defense advice needs to be active and actionable, meaning that it must compel and motivate us to do something new, preferably a something new we are confident we can do. Harris's piece appears to be what reasonable people might find reasonable about conflict advice, and that's exactly the problem—it fails to challenge us to change our perspective or our behavior. Instead, it soothes our vexation by supporting precisely what we would like to believe about ourselves, not what we need to know.

So much of martial experience is based on what folks perceive they want that it leads to wild misconceptions about what it can and will actually do for us. Any good marketing campaign not only showcases the product but also shapes and defines the buyer's need for it, a need that most might not have recognized they had. We don't always see what it is that we need, and instead we come up with wants that are not always accurate or possible. This makes it more difficult to approach martial training with any reliable sense of what it can do. It is the job of teachers to offer their expertise, but they should also articulate the needs that students should find valuable enough to embrace themselves.

There are no rules, caveats, or heuristics—let alone three quaint principles—that one can simply concur with and adopt to avoid conflict or deal with it when we cannot. Intellectualism is not the clearest way to understand conflict defense and its ethics. The physical is a far greater method to intuit the instinctive nature of our moral and ethical inclinations. No level of experience can be reached in any professional endeavor unless we first place ourselves under the conditions of its potential success and then attempt it over and again, failing as often as one must in order to fail less.

The way forward is clear: if we wish to better respond to conflict, be it potential or actual, then we must change both our perspective and our behavior. There is no other way to accomplish this than training to perceive order from conflict's chaos, identify the predictable in its spontaneous nature, and capture opportunities for resolution in its often erratic and awkward attempts to harm us or others.

The Moral as Martial: Ingenuity

Taking the world as it is seems like a reasonable and easy thing to do. But more often than not, we do not. Usually we're too busy perceiving it as we'd like it to be.

From the way we live our days to the jobs we have and the relations we cultivate, we are so busy repurposing, remodeling, and redefining our world, we have scant time for reminders of its reality, thereby choosing to live in the world we want, not the world that is. It's just easier and cuts down on conflict between like-minded folks who have accepted this.

But reality does rear its head, like a beast from the depths—clearly out of our control—that breaks the surface of our world to astonish us often with its violence and horror. We normally afford it the same attentions as a sighting of Bigfoot, or a light in the sky that defies the laws of physics. Afterward, we act as though these are one-offs, shunning them as exceptions to the basic rules that we have decided regulate this world. We pretend they are not examples of realities out of our direct influence.

But, of course, those seeming exceptions to the rules *are the rules*, the ones that bear consequences for nonadherence. Nature breaks our understanding of our world all the time, and consequently it catches people off guard time and again. Sometimes this results in lessons learned, to be heeded the next time, and sometimes the outcome is so dire there is no next time. Training should reflect this.

Check out this quote from the *Maneuver Warfare Handbook*, by William S. Lind. The quote itself is by Colonel Michael D. Wyly, US Marine Corps, from the introduction to a lecture series on tactics he delivered to the Amphibious Warfare School in the 1981–82 school year. It is highly informative.

After he declares that the "fundamentals" of tactics are not "control measures" and "formats" (read, techniques), he defines fundamentals as "that which dealt with defeating the enemy. The answer to the question of what will work to undo the opposing force is what we must be searching for in tactics. . . . All else is peripheral."[10] He continues,

> First the student must learn to think creatively, to innovate, and to do the things that will most quickly seek out the enemy's weak spots and undo him. Learning to think in that fashion is fundamental. . . . Once these fundamentals are learned, that is, once the student has begun to think clearly about how best to undo his adversary, once he has been rewarded in the classroom or the field for creative thought, the careful weighing of alternatives and risks followed by boldness in decision-making, he will then be ready to study definitions, control measures and formats. He will grasp their meaning more rapidly, for he will have a context in which to place them. They will be more than words and symbols.
>
> When we teach tactics in the opposite order, that is, the mechanics ahead of the thinking, too often we produce, instead of soldiers, structured mechanics who find it difficult to think without rules. The art of war has no traffic with rules. Yet I have often seen students reject their best tactical ideas because they could not fit them into the format.[11]

Wyly cautions against becoming "structured mechanics who find it difficult to think without rules" (think "technique collectors," folks only interested in accruing knowledge for its own sake). Concentrating on when we should and should not act opens us to opportunities for the use of a variety of techniques. So we must make a concentrated effort to let go of "what to do." Turns out, there is no what to do, only our personal ethical bearing and "when" and "where" to act on it. It is this combination that naturally produces the "what" of the technique.

All martial training exists to some extent in an envisioned dream world of our discretion. In fact, we must use a dream world of sorts in order to incorporate truths as we understand them into the fictions we design and utilize as training scenarios so we might understand these truths more clearly. Everyone utilizes this, from the local taekwondo kids' class to the hardest-charging military special operator. Drills, sparring, tactical exercises, and even kata are all accomplished through the use of creative fiction, as it is amenable to the human mind and can make sense to us.

But whereas fiction is a matter of "might be," truth does not have to be believable; it simply is. Facing and enduring the "moment of truth" has more to do with adapting to its pace of change rather than apprehending the exceptionally bizarre or banal examples the human mind can concoct to wage conflict. These examples can dumbfound, rendering the moment unintelligible and protracting, even immobilizing, any response. Being confronted by a knife- or gun-wielding opponent is a dumbfounding moment—most folks will simply not believe it's happening to them. In 2014, Mutahir Rauf, an exchange student from Pakistan attending Loyola University, reached for what he thought was a toy gun when he was mugged here in Chicago mere blocks from campus. He was murdered for it.

This is one of the inherent issues with so-called realistic training—it's paradoxical: scenarios have to make sense or else no one could accomplish them. But in making scenarios sensible, we defy the validity of the actual, the authenticity of dumbfounding truth, by the very act of making sense of them. Thus, unless one is actually doing something real, like jumping out of airplanes or working with live ammunition, "realistic" training is always as fictional as any made-for-TV movie because only real is real.

Better to construct training to push students to adapt practiced skills and techniques to the stresses of constant change so as to learn how to make new and better decisions. This is consistent with new research at Johns Hopkins University that confirms that when the body performs repetition in creative ways, it learns earlier. A process called reconsolidation is said to modify existing memories when new knowledge is introduced. It is being heralded for its ability to strengthen motor skills for musicians and athletes, as well as for its uses in rehabilitation.

Ingenuity (*nin*genuity, if you want to be ninja about it) and the dream world can power further comprehension and enrich our understanding of the complexities of our given endeavors. Questions we formulate and ask in training not only reveal to us new answers but also do something even more valuable: provide us the analogical insight to forge better questions. This is parallelism at work and is the underlying strength of the parable, the analogy, of training by context.

The English writer Hilaire Belloc said, "Parallelism consists in the illustration of some unperceived truth by its exact consonance with the reflection of a truth already known and perceived." We use parallelism to compare new people, experiences, and things with what we already know to decide their worth. In this regard, allegory is the most common method humans use to interpret and make sense of their world. Allegory allows us to connect instinctively to the essential care and protection of what we already value and creates a scale to weigh what we know or feel to be true against the unknown and unfamiliar. The ability to interpret life through analogy, to parallel different moments and treat them as extended metaphors, produces the kind of wisdom that has often kept humanity alive.

The power to parallel our feelings from one issue to another is most apparent in the first world in the outrage generated by feelings of injustice most often stoked by the bitter, simple-headed angst of social media, an arena where logic and reason can only compete in a no-good, unemployable brother-in-law kind of way.

Logic requires intellectual balance, adherence to its rules, and use of its special lexicon to achieve results. Logic has the power to prove, and it makes its case in the same way that a tailor constructs a suit that is expertly fitted to the body. But logic's work comes well after allegory has already convinced us we ought to be clothed to traverse the world. Allegory appeals to instinct and the emotive, the same lifeblood of art and passion that forsakes logic to climb Everest and rejects Cartesian philosophy in Romeo's overtures to Juliet, which surely would have quenched her fire faster than Friar Laurence wooing her in Greek.

I submit that it is not through logic or deductive or inductive reasoning that one comes to know the martial way more clearly but through the body's means of the parallel, analogous, and allegorical. The logical can certainly tell us what to do and feeds the belief that enduring repetitive, idealized motor skills under sterile conditions is the best way to inculcate and master them as muscle memory. But reliance on this kind of training does not provide the deliberations to link the lessons in context so we can know how and when to actually apply them across the continuum of circumstances. This is the rub for much of martial training, as its defensive ability is meant and designed to be utilized under those ever-changing conditions, and never solely idealized for mere performance.

This drive to indoctrinate external techniques and master them as "second nature" is what so much of martial training is focused on. But this is to shine the wrong side of the coin and concentrate on the logical imitation of techniques when we ought to be perceiving the martial through the instincts of our "first nature." In this way we can establish an analogical parallel between what comes naturally *to us* and what we wish to be natural *for us*.

Philosophically speaking, if there is such a thing as a "second" nature, then there must be a "first," as second can only be second once it follows first. "Second nature" is what we can develop and train ourselves to be able to do "naturally," but that is not natural to us. Our "first nature" aspects are those that come to us naturally, that is, without requiring special training to use and understand them. I would argue that the principles of the martial way are in fact embedded in this first-nature understanding of the world and include our sense of equilibrium, acuity, and the timing of our motivations.

These exact sensations that allowed humans to hunt, survive, and sustain themselves are the same utilized for interpersonal combat, warfare, and the protection and defense of self and others. To establish a mature conception for the use of martial techniques involves perceiving second-nature knowledge through the lens of our first nature's inherent abilities.

Ingenuity in our training by context, analogy, and parallelism is one of the surest methods to sharpen and refine our natural abilities to apply techniques, tactics, and strategies found in the lineages of bygone or contemporary martial arts.

Take the World as It Is

When Bruno Nunes, a thirty-seven-year-old father of three, boarded a bus in Rio de Janeiro on June 20, 2015, he had no idea it would be the scene of his death. An armed mugger stormed it sometime afterward and began robbing the trapped passengers. Having been mugged twice before, the father and coach had had enough. The beefy, square-jawed Nunes, an instructor of Brazilian jiujitsu (BJJ), approached from behind and, by all accounts, applied a "rear naked choke" to the gunman, hoping to end the attack.

But something went wrong. Nunes wound up shot just above his left eye, perhaps when the mugger aimed behind his head and fired.

If one were searching for the best martial arts training for self-and-others protection and defense, it might seem prudent to discard BJJ based on this story, or any of the other public failures that have left BJJ proponents wounded or dead—there have been several caught on video. Here was, by all rights, an expert in his field, a coach and teacher in Rio—its hometown, no less. Surely the fact that he failed to disarm a lone gunman, with surprise and the rear position to his advantage, attests to the weakness of training inherent in BJJ as a system of self-defense.

It would be easy to make this argument. But it would be wrong to make it.

There have been many other instances in which BJJ proponents have used their training to end real-world violence and conflict. It would be unfair to consider only the failures and none of these successes. In assessing stories, aggregation would be the way to go. Weighing the batch would then point us toward one side of the scale over the other, and, due to its popularity and ubiquity, there have been far more wins than losses.

But aggregation is problematic. These same stories of success and failure, of surviving or dying under stress, could be told about every studyable martial art in the world and, for that matter, no martial art whatsoever. In fact, there have been plenty more completely untrained people who have engaged violence and conflict with the very same outcomes as those described here. With this perspective, there is no sense to be made from it. It's akin to searching for the best religion and being swayed simply by the subjective stories of one group over another. Hardly the manner in which to best seek out spiritual clarity.

However, anecdotally is exactly how most folks enter into their choice for martial training, akin to any market-based decision, such as buying stereo equipment. They'll research what others have to say on the matter, they'll listen to their stories, and due diligence will inform what is most popular, fashionable, highly reviewed, and recommended. And then they will make choices, accepting in large measure the conclusions of groupthink.

Admittedly, paging through reviews is a decent way to buy a stereo. But this is a manufactured thing, in which every customer receives the exact same thing. Martial training is a method to achieve an intuited ideal, and it is activated by its user to become capable and worthwhile. And there are no warranties that it will.

People in conflict make both smart and poor decisions. Trained or untrained, experienced or not, some survive, still others do not. These stories unfold under stress, which is anything but predictable, and are simply what they are: anecdotes of people in conflict. None of these stories is about martial art itself, and none provides us insight into how good any one art may be, its training, or its resiliency. As such, they are not helpful as signposts pointing us toward any correct course.

To discover the best martial arts training for self-and-others protection and defense, we need not heed the protestations regarding any one particular form; we merely need to replicate the method the sporting world followed to achieve their mixed martial arts (MMA) form, the only form now used in competitive martial sports.

On November 12, 1993, the first Ultimate Fighting Championship (UFC) was held in Denver, Colorado, to a sitting audience of about 7,800 fans, with 80,000 more folks watching at home. Its premise was simple: battle for the title of most effective martial art.

Like a real-life *Enter the Dragon* or *Bloodsport*, by gathering a range of experts from their respective styles and facing them off in the ring, the championship was about to allow America to witness as unique a contest as any before. Boxing versus jiujitsu, savate versus sumo, wrestling versus karate—the fight card sounded like a casting call for the *Streetfighter* video game series, but it was all real—the fights, the stakes, the consequences. Who would win? And which art would be crowned lord of the ring?

But as Dave Meltzer of Yahoo Sports wrote, UFC1, as it would later be known, was mainly produced and directed by the famous BJJ Gracie family to highlight themselves and one of their youngest and most prominent sons, Royce, who would become champion of that first tournament and more later.[12] Little did anyone guess at the time that mainly inexperienced fighters had been handpicked by Royce's big brother Rorion to ensure Royce's best chances of success in the ring, now known as the "octagon," per its shape.

Nevertheless, the UFC series started a movement within the martial sports community to match the success of the lean and wily Gracie BJJ and even try to overcome its seemingly unstoppable effectiveness. And it would. In fact, several years later, even the unbeaten Royce was bested in the ring by "shoot wrestling," a hybrid style employed by a Japanese named Sakuraba, who later took the nickname "the Gracie Killer," for the number of wins he accrued over direct members of the family.

Members of the martial sports community at large were learning and absorbing everything they thought necessary and worthwhile to take into the octagon to dominate. And their guiding premise was this: *take the ring as it is.*

Those early limitations of the styles themselves were exactly why previous competitors had failed. Those who specialized in only one area now risked being beaten by those who were more generalized in their options. And so it was to the generalists and their simple approach of including the widest array of possibilities that we see where the sport has taken itself today.

The ring, the octagon, the sphere of competition itself was now the guiding light clarifying how competitors would shape, craft, and refine their fight. This meant maximizing every potential that the ring would bear according to the allowances and rules of the sport as it evolved. UFC1 was touted with only three rules: no biting, no eye gouging, and no groin attacks. Since then, the list of rules has grown exponentially to exclude head butts, glove grabs, small-joint manipulation, hair pulling, fish hooking, throat strikes, and clawing, pinching, or twisting the flesh.

The more limitations placed on variables competitors could not control, the greater the predictability for fighters because one now had foreknowledge of and potential influence over the actions of one's opponent, opening more avenues for idealized techniques to be created and utilized. For example, if glove grabs were disallowed, competitors were then free to craft tactics that led with gloves, placing them in normally direct peril but knowing that opponent defenses would not and could not, according to new rules, act against them. This made, at least in part, for a more predictive fight, and contestants could plan more diligently, and even fine-tune their training accordingly. The "real fight" spontaneity and visceral nature of the clash of dissimilar fighting cultures in the original matches was soon left far behind for uniform and refined technical expertise.

MMA is now a science of grappling, striking, kicking, and distinctive skill sets housed in each budding competitor. To forgo training in one skill in favor of another is to cede advantage to an opponent who may not have taken that chance. No serious competitor is now studying only one art, one style, or one method. Instead, everybody trains in everything. By calibrating training to all the available options afforded in the highly regulated and rule-based ring, MMA refined itself into an idealized style that plays to the strengths of each of its players just inside of a dozen years or so.

Does this mean, then, that MMA is the best martial arts training for self-and-others protection and defense? Is it the premiere method to best activate and physically articulate the protector ethic?

I do not believe so.

In fact, what it has become is indicative of exactly why I would not rely on it.

Only Real Is Real

To focus and rely on MMA to best provide the training to exemplify the protector ethic would break the cardinal point of MMA's endeavor, which was to take *the ring* as its guiding standard so it could embody all of the idealized techniques *competition* could give way to.

Self-and-others protection and defense does not occur in a ring, under competition, or with any set of rules or regulations. A life-and-death struggle is about survival and occurs instead in the real world. Thus, we must cede to that singular principle and recognize that there is no competitive martial sport that allows for the world as it is. Were this the case, the deficiencies of the training methods would become shockingly apparent, since they do not regularly train to instill a mind-set that accounts for real-world variables under normal training conditions. The default mind-set of martial sports is idealization and controlled competition, always and every time. The moral of this story is stark: perception is reality—*the way we perceive our training is the way we will train to perceive its use.*

How we perceive our training directly influences how we will train to perceive its use in the real world, and that goes for its ethics as well. Ring fighters are trained to think how to win in controlled conditions; protectors are trained to think how to protect and defend under ever-changing uncertainty. These radically different fundamental values account for why the training of these two perspectives is and ought to be distinct.

Martial sports are not defined by, do not inherently train for, do not intrinsically deal with, and are not expected to deal with the range of variable threats under conditions of life or death. There are folks who think that BJJ is the best way to test ground fighting, judo the best way to test throwing, and kendo the best way to test sword fighting. But to what end? For viability in the martial way to protect and defend life, I disagree on all counts. BJJ is best for tournament ground fighting, judo best for tournament throwing, and kendo best for tournament kendo because the manner of their training habituates their practitioners to perceive and utilize their techniques under those ideal, tournament conditions.

Judoka don't have to worry about getting stabbed by a used needle from a meth head in regular training, BJJitsuka don't have to worry about multiple attackers beating their skulls in with bats in regular training, and kendoka don't have to worry about their swords bending or breaking when they clash in regular training. If they did, if every iteration of their training concerned these aspects, if the very notion of their training was embedded and infused with such possibilities, their training as we know it today could not be their training because the idealization with which it is currently carried out cannot exist in a world with meth heads and their needles, multiple opponents and their bats, and swords that bend and break on impact.

None of their training would exist because none of it could exist in the context of surviving, protecting, and defending life. It only ever exists under controlled conditions—variable threats of the world be damned. Imagine a baseball player training to hit a fast pitch and then trying to do the same while concerning himself with the potential that the umpire, or the catcher, or both will set on him with stabbing weapons until he dies. If that possibility were an actual part of baseball proper, you wouldn't see baseball anymore, as it would morph into a life-protecting endeavor completely different from America's pastime.

I have great respect for those who train in competitive martial sports, as they are difficult and the training is all consuming. But it would be a lie to say principles of the martial way are used equivalently in defending a title and defending life. Though there will always be some overlap in all martial endeavors, there can be no true equivalence between sport and warrior arts—the two are mutually exclusive and must be. If martial sport adopted the same manner necessary for great ability in warrior arts, competition would stifle and by all measure become impractical as practitioners lured each other into possible career-ending outcomes, not to mention death. This manner would never allow any purely refined form or technique to take shape and flourish as it can and does under the highly controlled and regulated conditions of competition.

And if warrior arts adopted the manner of sport, practitioners would not learn foremost to close off any and all openings and vulnerabilities, since the performance of techniques would be all consuming, no matter the circumstances of their use. Just page through any book of judo or competition jiujitsu—its basic techniques have all been chosen, designed even, specifically for use in the strict two-person contest model. But this model fails the moment it takes into account any outside variables that make technical performance impractical and dangerous to the user, such as when makeshift weapons, multiple opponents, environmental dangers, and attack by ambush are considered—all of which are just a few of the most prominent issues in normal warrior art training.

Warriorship tries to attain a viable perspective that engenders a life-protecting ethic for self and others. It is this viability in training that directly shapes the habits of its principles into a broad, creative, asymmetric, and technically unconventional arsenal to protect life—points and winning notwithstanding. Strategy and tactics are also mirrored by situational awareness, clever use of the environment, and cunning manipulation through timing for the purposes of escape, intervention for the defense of others, or confrontation of enemies to be killed or, most dangerously, subdued for arrest or confinement.

Martial competition occurs between willing participants who normally assign similar value to tests of will, camaraderie, and fraternity. But getting home to one's family or protecting them or oneself through violent struggle is not and cannot be considered any game. There is only dealing with the violence of aggression and how well one survives it. Getting out ahead of such violence through awareness and avoidance, or adapting effectively to the least necessary outcome based on one's conditions and context, *this alone* marks such a major difference between sport and warrior training methods and perception of those methods that it in itself is enough to settle the stark difference.

Don't get me wrong, I'm not talking down any of these sports. They can be fun and exciting and provide worthwhile time spent with like-minded others for a plethora of good reasons. But one of those reasons is not reliance on them for the betterment of warrior arts—the context is too different. I would also not advocate warrior arts for the ring and for the same reason—when we assume the context is the same, because some of the techniques are, we wind up confused. There's a reason Michael Jordan didn't cut it as a baseball player after he retired from basketball. As wise as he was in the one case, he was not equally wise in the other. Why not? Because the ball playing was from a completely different context.

The reality of the world and the variable means by which the violent bring violence usually have little to do with how understandable it is to us, with how much it "makes sense." In fact, psychologically, interpersonal violence often confounds, which is why most people want no part of it. If it did make sense, training to counter and defend against it would be a hell of a lot easier than it is. But in the world as it actually is, not as we want or wish it to be, the only thing realistic is reality. *Only real is real.* Period. All our training, everyone's training, is a well-crafted fiction, and it must be for us to gain any understanding of extemporaneous viable change under variable conditions.

I often say there is no such thing as "realistic" training. Training is a fabrication we produce for ourselves in order to account for the fundamental aspects that are always present in reality—change and its variables. There is no training scenario that anyone could ever craft to mimic reality; there are simply too many impossibly strange variables and conditions to account for. Oh sure, some try by incorporating more variables, or raising the stress level, or crafting reenactments of true-life situations. But this can only ever be a high-stress production—a tactical play put on by willing performers. Only real is real: no one ever tries to kill you in training, and if they did, it would not be training; it would be real, and training ideals such as learning to habituate new and better tactics, applications, awareness, and overall behavior would not apply.

Context matters. It calibrates, directs, and helps us navigate untenable waters and thus permeates martial endeavor. And it matters so much, it is such an enormous part of what we do and how we are able to do it, that we often overlook it without thinking twice. Like any necessary aspect of our daily existence, like stable ground before an earthquake or breathable air, it is something that we only appreciate after it's become short in supply.

On the surface, there is always much in common between longtime actors of the martial ways. All of us are engaged in a process that changes us fundamentally and hopefully for the better. But when we dig into the details of our respective backgrounds, we inevitably find many differences in our training values. These differences ought not be compared ad nauseam but rather celebrated!

We ought to revel in the ability, sheer will, and technical expertise required to attain such advanced levels of pure martial ideal in the sporting world. And we should treat with all sacredness the wisdom and clarity that the ancient touchstone of humanity's protector ethic imbues us with to temper ourselves to stand up for, save, and defend the lives of ourselves and others in the crucible of human conflict.

Rectitude

The terrifying little reason why the virtue of courage and its steadfast reliance for rectitude is so important, and why physical training to enhance it is a must, is this: The opposite of courage is not cowardice, and it's not foolhardiness either. It's *appeasement*.

Courage, cowardice, and foolhardiness sit on a spectrum within the Aristotelian model. Under incredible stress, such as war, or the chaos of a savage nightclub shooting, someone might experience all three of these instincts in a span of moments. But appeasement is the willing act to perhaps sacrifice others to save oneself. This is uncut and pure nihilism: to give in and give up on truth in morality is to make sacrifices of others to save your own skin, an ultimately selfish act in that one refuses to protect others because that would mean risking oneself to do so in conflict. And that is simply too terrifying an act.

People who disregard truth will eventually be run over by it. These are the same folks who want to live their lives consequence-free and rail against self-reliance and self-and-others defense. Placing the responsibility for personal safety on everyone else, including authorities, isn't clear-headed and is certainly not serious reasoning. Nature—both mother and human—gets a vote too. And nature always votes for itself and wins every time. Jump off a building so you can fly and you'll fly right up until you hit the ground. It'll be a quick lesson about how much of your life is consequence-free.

Mother Nature does not have our best interests at heart. Neither does human nature. That's the truth. Alligators work hard at alligatoring. If you don't believe me, try petting one in the wild. Nature is defined by what it does, not by what we expect or want it to do. If we decide not to acknowledge this difference, or, worse, lie about it, then we remain ignorant of or dishonest about our duty to prevent alligators from alligatoring us.

If we do not or will not face the world as it is, then we're trapped by our own victimhood, where we continually refuse to acknowledge the essence of the issue—bad people do bad things, and that's why they are bad. This point is so frightening to so many because it burdens with a set of personal responsibilities many would rather ignore. It means we have to deal with the terrifying specter of conflict.

On a soulful level, we want to solve the problem of moral evil, though it is irresolvable. And since we cannot, many have found ways to protect themselves from the chaos of human nature, not by observation, recognition, and preparation of threats and dangers but by redefining their reality and stripping objectivity and absolutism from the objective and absolute. Evil is an objective reality—it exists. Evil is also an absolute certainty—it will always occur.

But when we decide to stop discriminating between better and best, good and not good, worse and worst, we arm ourselves not with any functioning defensive tool but with a rubber gun. When sickening attacks on innocents occur, we can invoke more authoritative politics to devalue and even disgrace the personal obligations we have toward each other. Our individual roles diminish as state-sponsored roles increase in power, making it all too easy to pass laws to keep people "safe."

This is why evil, as both a useful term and a deep concept, is so incredibly practical. Evil is a perfected ideal, one that cannot be and should not ever be ignored or taken for granted—it will surely not do that with you. We should be taught and teach others to fight against its inception and, when not fighting it, highlight its existence, be it systemic or nascent, endorsed or tacit.

But if we refuse, if we instead choose willful ignorance of and intellectual dishonesty regarding the banality of evil that affects everyone, then we will have refrained from telling the difference between the likes of right and wrong, since we will have already absolved ourselves of the difference between good and evil. We will have become more than cowards; we will have become appeasers, henchmen to evil itself. Winston Churchill, that British bulldog said, "An appeaser is one who feeds a crocodile hoping it will eat him last." What Churchill failed to mention is that appeasers will serve up everyone else first before succumbing themselves. Appeasement is never a plan for survival—it's a suicide note with the date to be written in.

Evil issues us a bold challenge: either we stand and face it or we turn our back. I vote to stand. So, like a vampire that keeps rising from the dead, moral relativism—that twisted goon in service to its nihilistic master—is disorientation from truth. Stake it through its heart, festoon it with garlic, coffinate, and rebury it in consecrated earth.

The sad truth is that eventually the stakes will rot and the garlic weaken. And the seductive forces of subjectivity offering protection and defense from the reality of the world will reconstitute.

Warriors temper themselves against the anvil of conflict. They become physically skilled in order to see themselves and others more justly. They willingly risk themselves to identify moral choices. They protect the sacred in making ethical decisions. And they stand in the face of evil, in spite of the dread they may feel, so they can be more consistent at courageous doing.

To attain rectitude for the protector ethic, constancy of courage strengthens one's character by feeling, thinking, and acting according to what the martial way informs us is inescapably, universally, and unquestioningly worthwhile: *being human is to have values, but valuing human being is to know what is essential to feeling, thinking, and acting on them ethically.*

NOTES

1. "Fearful, Frigid Night on Chicago's Lake Shore Drive," NBCNews.com, February 2, 2011, accessed October 23, 2017, http://www.nbcnews.com /id/41394461/ns/weather/t/fearful-frigid-night-chicagos-lake-shore-drive /#.We587VuPKpo.
2. Friedrich Wilhelm Nietzsche and Walter Kaufmann, *Basic Writings of Nietzsche: Birth of Tragedy: Beyond Good and Evil: On the Genealogy of Morals: Ecce Homo* (New York: Modern Library, 1968), 276.
3. "Intentional and gratuitous infliction of harm for its own sake, perpetrated by a villain who is malevolent to the bone, inflicted on a victim who is innocent and good." Steven Pinker, *The Better Angels of Our Nature: Why Violence Has Declined* (New York: Penguin Books, 2012), 496.
4. Ibid., 496.
5. Dave Grossman and Loren W. Christensen, *On Combat: The Psychology and Physiology of Deadly Conflict in War and in Peace* (Mascoutah, IL: Warrior Science Publications, 2008), 3.
6. Phillip Cole, *The Myth of Evil* (Edinburgh: Edinburgh University Press, 2006), 236.
7. John Kekes, *Facing Evil* (Princeton, NJ: Princeton University Press, 1990), 232.
8. Sam Harris, "The Truth about Violence," *Sam Harris* (blog), November 5, 2011, https://www.samharris.org/blog/item/the-truth-about-violence.
9. David Grossman, *On Killing: The Psychological Cost of Learning to Kill in War and Society* (Boston: Back Bay Books, 1996).
10. Quoted in William S. Lind, *Maneuver Warfare Handbook* (Boulder, CO: Westview, 1985), 72.
11. Ibid., 72.
12. Dave Meltzer, "First UFC Forever Altered Combat Sports," *Yahoo! Sports*, November 12, 2007, https://www.yahoo.com/news/first-ufc-forever -altered-combat-174700529--mma.html.

Epilogue

ON A LAZY TUESDAY AFTERNOON, a cool day in October, seventy-five-year-old James Vernon stops teaching chess so he can have a knife fight.

The retiree leads a weekly club for home-schooled kids at his town's library in Morton, Illinois. Violence is rare in the Pumpkin Capital of the World, where the sleepy village, two hours west of Chicago, is better known for the thousands of acres dedicated to the local Nestlé plant that cans up Libby's Pureed Pumpkin. Vernon has just finished a tutorial and the kids are squaring off when a pudgy man in glasses enters and screams, "I'm going to kill some people!" He's holding two big knives and blocks any exit. Startled, Vernon at first thinks it's a prank. He begins talking, trying to reason with the intruder. It doesn't work.

"But I did deflect his attention and calmed him a bit," Vernon said. "I asked him if he was from Morton, did he go to high school. I asked what his problem was. He said his life sucks. That's a quote."[1] Dustin Brown, anxiously clutching two five-inch blades, isn't kidding; his life does suck.

The nineteen-year-old is facing twenty-two separate counts for possession of child pornography. He'd been charged in March after investigators, tipped off by an online cache service, descended on him. When his high school discovered he'd been using their Internet to store files of prepubescent girls being raped, they expelled him. Brown is currently free on a $125,000 bond and his court date is just days away. If convicted, he'll likely join his brother, another winner, already incarcerated for molesting a minor.

Though hardly a Bond villain, Brown's plan is no less brutal. Over the last two weeks, he's convinced himself to stab as many children as he can before ending himself in similar fashion. When he storms his town's library at 3:25 p.m., he's already taped up the handles of a pair of hunting knives and slipped on grippy gloves, all to ensure his hold amid the gore he's likely to be covered with. When he sees the club's sixteen kids, some as young as seven, his infatuation with their torture turns his hate to bloodlust.

In those first moments, Vernon puts himself between Brown and the kids. The young killer is cutting himself, slicing into his left arm in a bid to scare, and that it does. But it also indicates he's right-handed, telling Vernon any attack is likely to begin there. He would later say his army hand-to-hand combat training, received some fifty years prior, came flooding back, specifically the lessons on fighting a knife—"Be fast and vigorous," it reminded him. So he takes a chance and steps toward Brown, who backs off. He takes another, with the same effect. This is the opening he needs to cue the kids to run, and they run like hell—out of the room, out of the library, and into the arms of their waiting mothers.

That's it for Brown. His sick obsession has spun his life out of control, and now he's lost the one chance to kill for it. In the last decision he makes as a free man, he's going to make this old man pay.

Brown moves on Vernon and stabs at his face, but the elder is quick, and his left hand takes the hit, carving through the webbing. There's an explosion of blood as an artery and tendon of his ring finger are severed.

But Vernon is not done. His right catches a necklace around the boy's neck and he jerks it hard. Brown lurches as his head snaps back, and Vernon sinks a knee into the kid's groin. Being the larger of the two, he spins, sweeping Brown onto the table as kings, queens, and pawns scatter to the floor. By the grace of God, Brown's left arm is pinned underneath him when he lands—knife and all—and Vernon's weight keeps it there, more than likely saving his life. Despite the wound, Vernon grabs Brown's free wrist and hammers his collarbone with his right. It's enough—Brown's arms go numb and he drops the knives. A librarian snatches up the blades and helps Vernon hold Brown until police arrive minutes later. The battle has lasted ninety seconds.

Vernon, a retired computer architect and military veteran who never served in combat, is rushed to the hospital and spends more than two hours in surgery to repair the damage. Dustin Brown is despondent. As they lead him from his final defeat, he tells the arresting officer, "I failed my mission to kill everyone." Vernon, though recovering, is back at chess club the following week.

An interviewer later asked him for his thoughts in those critical moments. He replied, "This can't happen here and I'm not going to let it happen. These kids are my responsibility right now."

NOTES

1. "Illinois Army Vet, 75, Saves 16 Kids from Knife-Wielding Teen Reportedly Plotting Mass Murder," Fox News, accessed October 24, 2017, http://www .foxnews.com/us/2015/10/16/illinois-army-vet-75-saves-16-kids-from -knife-wielding-teen-plotting-mass.html.

Acknowledgments

THIS WORK WOULD NOT HAVE been possible if not for the ceaseless efforts of several people.

My deepest thanks to my publisher, David Ripianzi of YMAA Publication Center, for taking a chance on me and my ideas. To my editor, T. G. LaFredo, whose great patience, drive, and expertise made my voice stronger, and made me a better writer. To my mentor, teacher, and friend, Jack Hoban, for his honesty in keeping my compass aligned. To my many friends, who both read and critiqued the work at various stages. To my mother and father who have never given up on their son the writer. To my wife, whose love and support knows no bounds.

And finally, my martial journey would not have been possible if not for my teachers, who shaped and inspired me. Dr. Masaaki Hatsumi revealed how to connect to the ageless sense of warriorship that both protects and defends our humanity. And Toshiro Nagato showed me a natural way to embody it.

My deepest gratitude to you all.

Works Cited

Aquinas, Thomas. *The Ethics of Aquinas*. Edited by Stephen J. Pope. Washington, DC: Georgetown University Press, 2002.

Aristotle. *Nicomachean Ethics*. Edited by Martin Ostwald. Upper Saddle River, NJ: Prentice Hall, 1999.

Armstrong, Ari. "Spock's Illogic: 'The Needs of the Many Outweigh the Needs of the Few.'" *The Objective Standard*, September 12, 2013. https://www.theobjectivestandard.com/2013/09/spocks-illogic-the-needs-of-the-many-outweigh-the-needs-of-the-few/.

Ashford, Elizabeth, and Tim Mulgan. "Contractualism." *The Stanford Encyclopedia of Philosophy*, fall 2012 ed., edited by Edward N. Zalta. https://plato.stanford.edu/archives/fall2012/entries/contractualism/.

Babwin, Don, and Lindsey Tanner. "A Fearful, Frigid Night on Iconic Chicago Road." Associated Press, February 2, 2011.

Brooks, David. "Let's All Feel Superior." *New York Times*, November 14, 2011.

Burke, Edmund. *The Works of the Right Honorable Edmund Burke*. Rev. ed. Vol. 5. Boston: Little, Brown, 1866.

Cole, Phillip. *The Myth of Evil*. Edinburgh: Edinburgh University Press, 2006.

Dvorak, Petula. "Passengers Watched Killing on Metro Car. Should They Have Intervened?" *The Washington Post*, July 9, 2015, accessed September 25, 2017. www.highbeam.com/doc/1P2-38500002.html?refid=easy_hf.

Finley, M. I. *The World of Odysseus*. Introduction by Simon Hornblower. London: Folio Society, 2002.

Fleming, Ian. *You Only Live Twice*. New York: Penguin, 2003.

Friedfeld, Oliver. "I Was Mugged, and I Understand Why." *Hoya*, November 18, 2014. http://www.thehoya.com/i-was-mugged-and-i-understand-why/.

Funakoshi, Gichin, and Genwa Nakasone. *The Twenty Guiding Principles of Karate*. Tokyo: Kodansha International, 2008.

Glover, Jonathan. *Humanity: A Moral History of the Twentieth Century*. New Haven, CT: Yale University Press, 1999.

Gowans, Chris. "Moral Relativism." *The Stanford Encyclopedia of Philosophy*, winter 2016 ed., edited by Edward N. Zalta. https://plato.stanford.edu/archives/win2016/entries/moral-relativism/.

Graham, Gordon. *Theories of Ethics*. New York: Routledge, 2011.

Grossman, Dave. *On Killing: The Psychological Cost of Learning to Kill in War and Society*. Boston: Back Bay Books, 1996.

Grossman, Dave, and Loren W. Christensen. *On Combat: The Psychology and Physiology of Deadly Conflict in War and in Peace*. Mascoutah, IL: Warrior Science Publications, 2008.

Harris, Sam. "The Truth about Violence." *Sam Harris* (blog), November 5, 2011. https://www.samharris.org/blog/item/the-truth-about-violence.

Hoban, Jack. *The Ethical Warrior*. Spring Lake, NJ: RGI Media and Publications, 2012.

The Holy Bible: Containing the Old and New Testaments. New York: American Bible Society, 1986.

Humphrey, Robert L. *Values for a New Millennium*. Maynardville, TN: Life Values, 2005.

Kant, Immanuel. *Groundwork for the Metaphysics of Morals*. Translated by Mary Gregor. New York: Cambridge University Press, 2007.

Keegan, John. *A History of Warfare*. New York: Vintage Books, 1994.

Kekes, John. *Facing Evil*. Princeton, NJ: Princeton University Press, 1990.

Kluckhohn, Clyde. *Mirror for Man: The Relation of Anthropology to Modern Life*. London: George G. Harrap, 1950.

Lind, William S. *Maneuver Warfare Handbook*. Boulder, CO: Westview, 1985.

Meltzer, Dave. "First UFC Forever Altered Combat Sports." *Yahoo! Sports*, November 12, 2007. https://www.yahoo.com/news/first-ufc-forever-altered-combat-174700529--mma.html.

Nevius, C. W. "Veterans Share Views on Iraq War." *SFGATE*, December 13, 2005.

Nickerson, Raymond. "Confirmation Bias: A Ubiquitous Phenomenon in Many Guises." *Review of General Psychology* 2, no. 2 (June 1998): 175–220.

Nietzsche, Friedrich Wilhelm, and Walter Kaufmann. *Basic Writings of Nietzsche: Birth of Tragedy: Beyond Good and Evil: On the Genealogy of Morals: Ecce Homo*. New York: Modern Library, 1968.

Petruso, Karl M. "Early Weights and Weighing in Egypt and the Indus Valley." *M Bulletin* (Museum of Fine Arts, Boston) 79 (1981): 44–51.

Pinker, Steven. *The Better Angels of Our Nature: Why Violence Has Declined.* New York: Penguin Books, 2012.

Rachels, James. *The Elements of Moral Philosophy.* 6th ed. Edited by Stuart Rachels. Boston: McGraw Hill, 2010.

Twain, Mark. *Plymouth Rock and the Pilgrims and Other Salutary Platform Opinions.* Edited by Charles Neider. New York: Harper and Row, 1984.

Ward, Maisie. *Gilbert Keith Chesterton.* Lanham, MD: Rowman & Littlefield, 2005.

About the Author

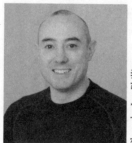

Photo by Jon Phillips

JAMES V. MORGANELLI has studied martial arts for forty years. His writing has appeared in *Black Belt* magazine. In 2001, his screenplay "Captive Moon" was a Finalist/Winner awarded by FilmMakers.com. A graduate of the University of Illinois at Urbana-Champaign, he majored in philosophy and held a concentration in East Asian languages and culture. In 2013, he received a master of arts in social philosophy from Loyola University Chicago, where he concentrated his studies on applied ethics and natural law. James has been certified in verbal defense and influence and is a master instructor in Bujinkan Budo Taijutsu of Japan, where he lived and trained for three years. Upon his return from Japan, he founded the Shingitai-Ichi Dojo in 1998 to continue his training, teaching, and outreach. James is also a staff member at Resolution Group International—professional conflict-resolution experts dedicated to teaching ethical, verbal, and physical skills to civilians, law enforcement, and the military. It is headed by Jack Hoban. James is also the founder and Director of the Protector Ethic Institute. Find more information at www.protectorethic.org. James lives in Chicago with his wife.

DVDS FROM YMAA

more products available from . . .
YMAA Publication Center, Inc. 楊氏東方文化出版中心
1-800-669-8892 • info@ymaa.com • www.ymaa.com